Melanonychias

Nilton Di Chiacchio • Antonella Tosti

Editors

Melanonychias

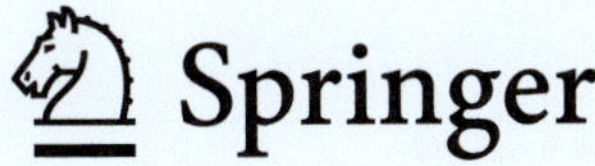 Springer

Editors
Nilton Di Chiacchio
Hospital do Servidor Público Municipal
São Paulo, São Paulo, Brazil

Antonella Tosti
University of Miami
Miami, Florida, USA

ISBN 978-3-319-83182-4   ISBN 978-3-319-44993-7   (eBook)
DOI 10.1007/978-3-319-44993-7

Printed on acid-free paper

This Springer imprint is published by Springer Nature
The registered company is Springer International Publishing AG
The registered company address is: Gewerbestrasse 11, 6330 Cham, Switzerland

Preface

Melanonychia can be caused by simple activation of the melanocytes of the nail matrix or by nonmalignant (nevi, lentigo) or malignant proliferation. Understanding and diagnosing melanonychia is still a challenge for general physicians and for dermatologists. The goal in the management of melanonychia is the early diagnosis of melanoma of the nail matrix and nail bed.

To improve the knowledge of melanonychia, a group of doctors with a special interest in nail diseases had several meetings to discuss diagnostic and management guidelines. The first meeting was held in San Antonio, Texas, in 2008, followed by others in Paris, Berlin, Miami, San Francisco, and New Orleans.

This book is the result of those meetings. All aspects of nail pigmentation are covered, from the characteristics and distribution of melanocytes in the normal nail to the histopathology of each lesion.

Readers learn the clinical and dermoscopic features that help the clinician in choosing lesions that should undergo excisional biopsy. Different treatment options are offered and discussed.

We hope that the book provides dermatologists and other doctors interested in nail pigmentation with the knowledge they need for optimal patient management (Fig. 1).

Miami, FL, USA — Antonella Tosti
São Paulo, São Paulo, Brazil — Nilton Di Chiacchio

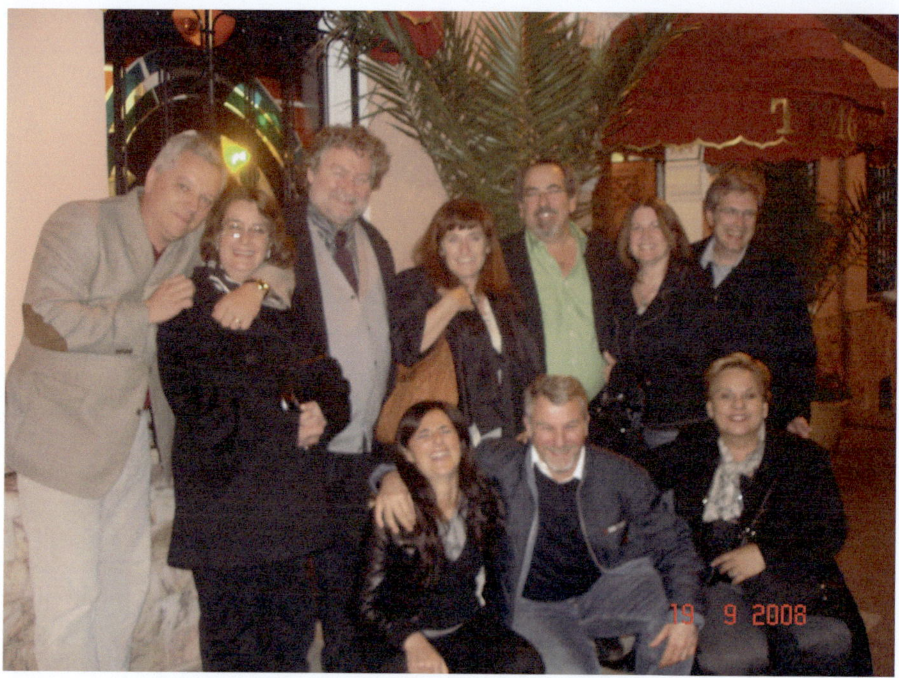

Fig. 1   Part of the International Group of Melanonychias, Paris, 2008

Contents

1 Melanocytes of the Nail 1
Lauren McCaffrey and Philip Fleckman

2 Epidemiology of Melanonychias 5
Beth S. Ruben and C. Ralph Daniel

**3 Clinical Evaluation: Clinical Features, Worrisome Signs,
and the ABCDEF Rule** 9
Shari R. Lipner and Richard K. Scher

4 Dermoscopy of the Nail Plate, Nail Matrix, and Nail Bed 25
Nilton Di Chiacchio, Diego L. Bet, and Nilton Gioia Di Chiacchio

5 Hypermelanosis (Melanocyte Activation) 45
Brian E. Bishop and Antonella Tosti

6 Lentigo and Nevus 57
Eckart Haneke

7 Subungual Melanoma 71
Judith Domínguez-Cherit, Daniela Gutiérrez-Mendoza,
Mariana de Anda-Juarez, Verónica Fonte-Avalos and
Sonia Toussaint-Caire

8 Melanonychia in Children 85
Bianca Maria Piraccini, Aurora Alessandrini, Emi Dika,
and Michela Starace

9 Non-melanocytic Melanonychia 97
Anna Q. Hare, Emily Bolton, and Phoebe Rich

**10 Histological Analysis of the Nail Plate in the Diagnosis of
Melanonychia and Other Nail Pigmentation** 111
Beth S. Ruben

11 Biopsy 119
Lucy Chen, Giselle Prado, and Martin Zaiac

12   Histopathological Analysis   131
Nilceo S. Michalany, Maria Victoria Suarez Restrepo, and
Leandro Fonseca Noriega

13   Treatment of Nail Unit Melanoma   141
Bertrand Richert

Index   151

Contributors

Aurora Alessandrini Department of Specialised Experimental and Diagnostic Medicine, Dermatology, University of Bologna, Bologna, Italy

Mariana de Anda-Juarez Hospital General "Dr Manuel Gea Gonzalez", México City, México

Diego L. Bet Hospital do Servidor Público Municipal, São Paulo, Brazil

Brian E. Bishop, BS Department of Dermatology and Cutaneous Surgery, University of Miami Leonard M. Miller School of Medicine, Miami, FL, USA

Emily Bolton, MS Creighton University School of Medicine, California Plaza, Omaha, NE, USA

Lucy Chen, MD Department of Dermatology and Cutaneous Surgery, University of Miami, Miami, United States

C. Ralph Daniel, MD Department of Dermatology, University of Mississippi Medical Center, Jackson, MS, USA

Nilton Di Chiacchio Hospital do Servidor Público Municipal, São Paulo, Brazil

Nilton Gioia Di Chiacchio Hospital do Servidor Público Municipal, São Paulo, Brazil

Medical School of ABC, São Paulo, Brazil

Judith Domínguez-Cherit Instituto Nacional de Ciencias Médicas y Nutrición Salvador Zubiran, Mexico City, Mexico

Emi Dika Department of Specialised Experimental and Diagnostic Medicine, Dermatology, University of Bologna, Bologna, Italy

Philip Fleckman, MD Dermatology, University of Washington, Seattle, WA, USA

Verónica Fonte-Avalos Hospital General "Dr Manuel Gea Gonzalez", México City, México

Daniela Gutiérrez-Mendoza Hospital General "Dr Manuel Gea Gonzalez", México City, México

Eckart Haneke, MD, PhD Department of Dermatology, Inselspital, University of Bern, Bern, Switzerland

Dermatology Practice Dermaticum, Freiburg, Germany

Centro Dermatol, Inst CUF, Porto, Portugal

Department of Dermatology, Academic Hospital, University of Gent, Ghent, Belgium

Anna Q. Hare, MD Department of Dermatology, Oregon Health and Science University, Portland, OR, USA

Shari R. Lipner, MD, PhD Weill Cornell Medicine and Dermatology, New York, NY, USA

Lauren McCaffrey, MD Dermatology, Group Health, Seattle, WA, USA

Nilceo S. Michalany, MD Departamento de Dermatologia, da Universidade Federal de, São Paulo, Brazil

Leandro Fonseca Noriega, MD Departamento de Dermatologia, Hospital do Servidor Publico Municipal, São Paulo, Brazil

Bianca Maria Piraccini Department of Specialised Experimental and Diagnostic Medicine, Dermatology, University of Bologna, Bologna, Italy

Giselle Prado, BS Herbert Wertheim College of Medicine, Florida International University, Miami, FL, United States

Maria Victoria Suarez Restrepo, MD Departamento de Dermatologia, Hospital do Servidor Publico Municipal, São Paulo, Brazil

Phoebe Rich, MD Department of Dermatology, Oregon Health and Science University, Portland, Oregon

Bertrand Richert, MD, PhD Dermatology Department, Brugmann – Saint Pierre – Queen Fabiola University Hospitals, Université Libre de Bruxelles, Brussels, Belgium

Beth S. Ruben, MD Department of Dermatology, University of California, San Francisco, CA, USA

Dermatopathology Service, Palo Alto Medical Foundation, Palo Alto, CA, USA

Richard K. Scher, MD, FACP Weill Cornell Medicine and Dermatology, New York, NY, USA

Michela Starace Dermatology, Department of Experimental, Diagnostic and Specialty Medicine, University of Bologna, Bologna, Italy

Antonella Tosti, MD Department of Dermatology and Cutaneous Surgery, University of Miami Leonard M. Miller School of Medicine, Miami, FL, USA

Sonia Toussaint-Caire Hospital General "Dr Manuel Gea Gonzalez", México City, México

Martin Zaiac, MD Director Greater Miami Skin and Laser Center, Mount Sinai Medical Center, Florida, United States

Melanocytes of the Nail

Lauren McCaffrey and Philip Fleckman

Key Features
- Melanocytes are present throughout the nail unit, including the matrix, nail bed, and hyponychium.
- The density of melanocytes is significantly lower in the nail unit than in other anatomical locations.
- Normal nail matrix melanocytes can be seen dispersed throughout the lower layers of the matrix epithelium.
- The proximal nail matrix contains a predominantly dormant population of melanocytes, whereas the distal matrix contains both dormant and active melanocyte populations.

Introduction

Melanocytes are a normal constituent cell population of the nail unit and can be found throughout all parts. There are, however, key differences between melanocytes of the nail unit and those of other anatomical areas. An understanding of melanocytes is critical for understanding the normal nail, and for differentiating benign causes of melanonychia from melanoma.

L. McCaffrey, MD
Dermatology, Group Health, Seattle, WA, USA

P. Fleckman, MD (✉)
Dermatology, University of Washington, Seattle, WA, USA
e-mail: fleck@uw.edu

© Springer International Publishing Switzerland 2017
N. Di Chiacchio, A. Tosti (eds.), *Melanonychias*,
DOI 10.1007/978-3-319-44993-7_1

History

Little was known about the melanocytes of the nail unit until 1968, when Higashi (1968) first demonstrated DOPA-positive melanocytes in the nail matrix. Shortly thereafter, Higashi and Saito (1969) demonstrated important differences between the density and distribution of melanocytes in the nail unit compared with melanocytes of normal skin. Further work by Tosti et al. (1994) clarified the immunohistochemical profile of melanocytes in the nail matrix, and Perrin et al. (1997) clarified the maturation and differentiation of melanocytes in the proximal and distal matrix. These important studies further informed the current understanding of nail matrix melanocytes. Since that time, ongoing study of nail matrix melanocytes has focused on differentiation between benign and malignant causes of longitudinal melanonychia.

Developments

Melanocytes are present throughout the epithelium of the nail apparatus, including the matrix, the nail bed, and the hyponychium. One study of nail unit melanocytes described the presence of small clusters of melanocytes present in normal nail matrix epithelium (Tosti et al. 1994), although this finding has not been duplicated. Thus, most authors consider singly-dispersed melanocytes to be the normal pattern in nail epithelium (Perrin et al. 1997). Melanocytes in the nail bed can be quantified by two different methods. The melanocyte count (MC) is defined as the number of melanocytes per millimeter of the dermoepidermal junction, as visualized on standard vertical histological sections (Amin et al. 2008). The density of melanocytes is measured as the number of melanocytes per square millimeter, as visualized on epidermal sheets prepared from nail matrix epithelium (Higashi and Saito 1969; Perrin et al. 1997). The average melanocyte count in the nail matrix is estimated to be between 4 and 20 melanocytes per millimeter of basement membrane length (Tosti et al. 1994; Amin et al. 2008; Perrin 2013), depending upon fixation and staining conditions. The density of matrix melanocytes in normal nail matrix has been estimated to range from ~100 to ~300 melanocytes per square millimeter (see below) (Higashi and Saito 1969; Perrin et al. 1997). There is some overlap between the MC of normal, nonpigmented nail (4–9/mm), and benign subungual lentigo, which has a reported MC between 5 and 31, and a grey zone between the upper level in subungual lentigo and the lower level in melanoma. However, the MC of normal nail is significantly lower than the reported MC in subungual melanoma in situ, which has been reported to range from 39 to 136/mm (Amin et al. 2008).

The relatively low density of melanocytes in the nail matrix contrasts with the higher melanocyte density seen in glabrous skin, which ranges from 500 to 4,500 melanocytes per mm^2 (Higashi and Saito 1969). Additionally, in contrast to glabrous skin, normal melanocytes of the nail matrix are commonly present in epidermal layers above the basal layer (Higashi 1968; Tosti et al. 1994). In the proximal matrix, where the matrix epithelial thickness is greatest (typically 8–10 layers), melanocytes can be demonstrated throughout the lower epithelial layers, including the superficial epithelium just below the keratogenous layers. The distal matrix typically measures only two to three cells thick, and here, melanocytes typically reside in the lowest two layers of the epithelium (Perrin et al. 1997). This more superficial location of melanocytes in the matrix epithelium should not be mistaken for pagetoid spread or evidence of malignancy. In the apical nail matrix, the hyponychium, and the nail bed, the typical basal location of melanocytes, is preserved (Perrin 2013). Why the distribution of melanocytes differs from that of other anatomical sites is unclear, but has been postulated to be related to the fact that the matrix has multiple layers of immature keratinocytes, or differences in the distribution of adhesion molecules in the nail matrix epithelium (Higashi 1968; Tosti et al. 1994).

On a cellular level, dendrites from nail matrix melanocytes extend in every direction, and when melanin pigment is present, the granules demonstrate a gradient of density, becoming more numerous in superficial layers of matrix epithelium, with aggregates of granules over keratinocyte nuclei (Higashi 1968). The distal matrix epithelium contains more numerous and larger melanocytes than the proximal matrix (Higashi and Saito 1969; Tosti et al. 1994). An ultrastructural study of normal nails showed that Caucasian nails have only rare discernable melanosomes. In this study, Asian subjects had more numerous melanosomes, with various stages of maturation, although most were in the immature stages. Specimens from African–American skin showed the most numerous melanosomes, which were mature and contained dense melanin pigmentation (Hashimoto 1971).

By staining for various melanosome-related proteins, melanocytes of the nail matrix can be further characterized. Tyrosinase-related protein-1 (TRP-1) is a protein that is restricted to early (stage I/II) melanosomes. L-DOPA is an enzyme present only in pigment-producing melanocytes, and its presence requires functional differentiation of the melanocyte. The proximal nail matrix contains melanocytes that are TRP-1-, but none that are L-DOPA-positive. Conversely, the distal nail matrix contains both melanocytes that are L-DOPA-positive, and those that are TRP-1-positive, which are slightly more numerous. The nail bed contains few melanocytes, and those that are present are TRP-1 positive. Thus, the proximal matrix contains predominantly dormant melanocytes, as does the nail bed, although the density in the nail bed is much lower. The distal matrix contains two populations of melanocytes: those that are functionally differentiated, and those that are dormant (Perrin et al. 1997). Thus, it is thought that longitudinal melanonychia related to melanocyte activation is derived from melanocytes of the distal matrix.

Additionally, nail melanocytes are uniformly marked with the monoclonal antibody HMB45, which recognizes a cytoplasmic antigen in the pre-melanosome. HMB45 typically marks fetal melanocytes, and can stain blue nevi and melanoma cells, but is not reactive with normal melanocytes of glabrous skin, in contrast to the staining pattern of normal nail matrix melanocytes (Tosti et al. 1994; Perrin et al. 1997). Like the unique distribution of nail matrix melanocytes, this should not be considered a finding worrisome for malignancy in the nail unit.

Outlook: Future Developments

Many advancements in our understanding of the melanocytes of the nail unit have occurred in recent decades. However, overlap with characteristics of malignant conditions – including the density of melanocytes, their superficial location in the epithelium, and staining with HMB45 – complicates differentiation between benign malignant melanocytic neoplasms of the nail unit. Further studies are necessary to characterize more completely the maturity, function, and staining patterns of normal matrix melanocytes to improve the diagnostic accuracy of such conditions.

Summary for the Clinician
Melanocytes are normally present throughout the nail unit, but lower in density than melanocytes of glabrous skin. Importantly, melanocytes in the nail matrix can be present throughout the layers of the matrix epithelium, which should not be confused with a malignant finding. The proximal nail matrix and nail bed contain populations of dormant melanocytes, whereas the distal matrix contains both dormant and mature pigment-producing melanocytes. Thus, distal matrix melanocytes are more likely to contribute to the formation of longitudinal melanonychia.

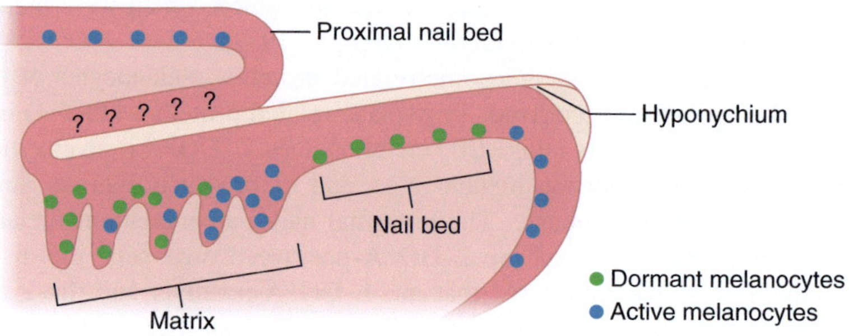

References

Amin B, Nehal KS, Jungbluth AA, Zaidi B, Brady MS, Coit DC, et al. Histologic distinction between subungual lentigo and melanoma. Am J Surg Pathol. 2008;32(6):835–43.
Hashimoto K. Ultrastructure of the human toenail. I. Proximal nail matrix. J Invest Dermatol. 1971;56(3):235–46.
Higashi N. Melanocytes of nail matrix and nail pigmentation. Arch Dermatol. 1968;97(5):570–4.
Higashi N, Saito T. Horizontal distribution of the dopa-positive melanocytes in the nail matrix. J Invest Dermatol. 1969;53(2):163–5.
Perrin C. Tumors of the nail unit. A review. Part I: acquired localized longitudinal melanonychia and erythronychia. Am J Dermatopathol. 2013;35(6):621–36.
Perrin C, Michiels JF, Pisani A, Ortonne JP. Anatomic distribution of melanocytes in normal nail unit: an immunohistochemical investigation. Am J Dermatopathol. 1997;19(5):462–7.
Tosti A, Cameli N, Piraccini BM, Fanti PA, Ortonne JP. Characterization of nail matrix melanocytes with anti-PEP1, anti-PEP8, TMH-1, and HMB-45 antibodies. J Am Acad Dermatol. 1994;31(2 Pt 1):193–6.

Epidemiology of Melanonychias

2

Beth S. Ruben and C. Ralph Daniel

> **Key Features**
> - Melanonychia may occur in all age groups.
> - Melanonychia is more common in adults than in children.
> - The peak age of incidence of nail unit melanoma is 50–70 years.
> - Nail unit melanocytic nevus with longitudinal melanonychia is more frequent in children than in adults.
> - African–Americans present a higher incidence of longitudinal melanonychia.
> - Nail unit melanoma is more common among all melanoma subtypes in dark-skinned persons.
> - Nail melanoma in children is rare.

Melanonychia is a type of nail dyschromia and occurs when nail apparatus melanocytes produce melanin pigment. The most common manifestation is longitudinal melanonychia (LM). In this case, the more active distal matrix melanocytes usually produce pigment, appearing most commonly in the deeper portion of the nail plate. However, the manifestations of melanonychia are protean and may affect almost any part of the nail unit. The apparent color change may appear black, brown, or grayish. Nail melanoma is often associated with LM, in roughly 75% of cases in some series.

Blackish and brownish nail pigment has many causes (Zaiac and Daniel 2005). Melanonychia may occur in all age groups. Congenital melanonychia may occur and can fade or darken over time (Thomas et al. 2012). It is most often due to a

B.S. Ruben, MD (✉)
Department of Dermatology, University of California, San Francisco, CA, USA

Dermatopathology Service, Palo Alto Medical Foundation, Palo Alto, CA, USA
e-mail: RubenBS@sutterhealth.org

C.R. Daniel, MD
Department of Dermatology, University of Mississippi Medical Center, Jackson, MS, USA

© Springer International Publishing Switzerland 2017
N. Di Chiacchio, A. Tosti (eds.), *Melanonychias*,
DOI 10.1007/978-3-319-44993-7_2

nevus (Thomas et al. 2012; Tosti and Piraccini 2009). In fact, some researchers proposed that LM in children does not require diagnostic biopsy, except for those lesions that rapidly increase in width and darkness (Abimelec and Dumantie 2005; Goettmann et al. 1999). LM is more common in adults than in children and it rarely occurs in children under the age of 10 (de Berker et al. 2012). The incidence of nail unit melanocytic nevus within LM has been recorded to be 22.5% in adults and 47.5% in children (Abimelec and Dumantie 2005; Goettmann et al. 1999). LM occurs in 77% of African–Americans over the age of 20 and the incidence is almost 100% over the age of 50 (Thomas et al. 2012). It occurs in 10–20% of Japanese people (Thomas et al. 2012).

Thumbs and index fingers are most frequently involved in African–Americans, and in Japanese, thumbs, index, and middle fingers (Thomas et al. 2012). Baran has called melanonychia related to physical contact and trauma "frictional melanonychia" (Thomas et al. 2012). Frictional melanonychia (Baran and Dawber 1994) is likely the most common cause of LM. It is also termed melanocytic activation or hypermelanosis, and has a variety of causes besides trauma, which are discussed elsewhere in this book. In general, it is more commonly seen in darker-skinned individuals and as age advances. Nail melanoma in children is rare and only three cases have been reported in fair skinned individuals (Tosti et al. 2005, 2012), Bonamonte and Arpaia, 2014). Thirteen cases have been reported in the literature, of which ten presented clinically as LM (Tosti et al. 2012). None has been invasive.

Larger-scale epidemiological studies of nail unit melanoma are needed, but some larger series have offered data on the prevalence and other characteristics (Haneke 2012; Banfield et al. 1998; Thai et al. 2001; Kato et al. 1996; O'Leary et al. 2000). In light-skinned white patients, 1.5–2% of all melanoma occur in the nail unit, whereas in dark-skinned patients over 20% of melanomas occur at this site. However, the overall absolute incidence is similar. The peak age of the incidence of nail unit melanoma is 50–70 years. Whether there is a gender preference remains unclear. The thumb and great toe are most often affected, followed by the index finger and the middle finger.

References

Abimelec P, Dumantie C. Basic and advanced nail surgery. In: Scher RK, Daniel RC, et al (eds) Nails: diagnosis, therapy, and surgery. 3rd ed. Philadelphia: Elsevier; 2005. p. 291–307.

Banfield CC, Redburn JC, Dawber RP. The incidence and prognosis of nail apparatus melanoma. A retrospective study of 105 patients in four English regions. Br J Dermatol. 1998;139(2): 276–9.

Baran R, Dawber RPR. Physical signs. In: Diseases of the nails and their management. 2nd ed. Oxford: Blackwell; 1994; p. 35–80.

Bonamonte D, Arpaia N. In situ melanoma of the nail unit presenting as a rapid growing melanonychia in a 9-year-old white boy. J Dermatol Surg. 2014;40(10):1154–7.

De Berker AR, Richert B, Baran R. The nail in childhood and old age. In: Baran R, de Berker DAR, Holzberg M, Thomas L, et al (eds) Baran and Dawber's diseases of the nails and their management. 4th ed. Oxford: Wiley; 2012. p. 183–209.

Goettmann S, Andre J, Belaich S. Longitudinal melanonychia in children. J Am Acad Dermatol. 1999;41:17–22.

Haneke E. Ungual melanoma – controversies in diagnosis and treatment. Dermatol Ther. 2012;25(6):510–24.

Kato T, Suetake T, Sugiyama Y, Tabata N, Tagami H. Epidemiology and prognosis of subungual melanoma in 34 Japanese patients. Br J Dermatol. 1996;134(3):383–7.

O'Leary JA, Berend KR, Johnson JL, Levin LS, Seigler HF. Subungual melanoma. A review of 93 cases with identification of prognostic variables. Clin Orthop Relat Res. 2000;378:206–12.

Thai KE, Young R, Sinclair RD. Nail apparatus melanoma. Australas J Dermatol. 2001;42(2): 71–81. quiz 82–83

Thomas L, Zook EG, Haneke E, et al. Tumors of the nail apparatus and adjacent tissues. In: Baran R, de Berker DAR, Holzberg M, Thomas L, et al (eds) Baran and Dawber's disease of the nails and their management. 4th ed. Oxford: Wiley; 2012. G370743.

Tosti A, Piraccini BM. Pediatric disease. In: Scher RK, Daniel RC, et al (eds) Nails, diagnosis, therapy surgery, 3rd ed.. Philadelphia: Elsevier; 2009. p. 229–243.

Tosti A, Piraccini BM, Cagalli A, Haneke E. In situ melanoma of the nail unit in children: report of two cases in fair skinned Caucasian children. Pediatr Dermatol. 2012;29:79–83.

Tosti A, Richert B, Pazzaglia M. Tumors of the nail apparatus. In: Scher RK, Daniel RC, et al (eds) Nails, diagnosis, therapy, surgery. 3rd ed. Philadelphia: Elsevier; 2005.

Zaiac M, Daniel C. Pigmentation abnormalities. In: Scher, Daniel, et al. (eds) Nails, diagnosis, therapy, surg. 3rd ed. Elsevier, Philadelphia. p. 73–90. 2005.

Clinical Evaluation: Clinical Features, Worrisome Signs, and the ABCDEF Rule

Shari R. Lipner and Richard K. Scher

Key Features
- Longitudinal melanonychia (LM) is defined as a vertical band of brown–black pigment that extends from the matrix to the distal portion of the nail plate.
- One of the most important diagnostic possibilities when evaluating LM is subungual melanoma, which carries a poor prognosis, although the survival rate is improved with early detection.
- Evaluation of LM starts with a thorough history of the pigmented nail band.
- The clinical examination should include evaluation of the color and width of the pigmentation in addition to the surrounding skin.
- The ABCDEF rule incorporates many of the key components of the history and clinical evaluation of LM and can be useful in the decision to biopsy for subungual melanoma.
- Histopathology remains the gold standard for the diagnosis of LM.

Introduction

Melanonychia means "black nail" and longitudinal melanonychia (LM), or melanonychia striata, refers to vertical bands of brown–black pigment that extend from the matrix to the distal portion of the nail plate. This brown–black color may be caused by exogenous pigment, infectious causes, or benign or malignant melanocytic etiologies. The most important diagnostic consideration when evaluating LM is

S.R. Lipner, MD, PhD (✉) • R.K. Scher, MD, FACP
Weill Cornell Medicine and Dermatology, New York, NY, USA
e-mail: shl9032@med.cornell.edu

© Springer International Publishing Switzerland 2017
N. Di Chiacchio, A. Tosti (eds.), *Melanonychias*,
DOI 10.1007/978-3-319-44993-7_3

subungual melanoma, which carries a poor prognosis compared with other cutaneous melanomas (Ruben 2010; Levit et al. 2000). This poor prognosis is partially attributed to more advanced disease as a result of delayed diagnosis (Levit et al. 2000; Quinn et al. 1996; English and Hammert 2012; Ilyas et al. 2012). As LM is seen in about two-thirds of nail melanomas (Ruben 2010; Haneke and Baran 2001), it is important for physicians to understand the proper examination of pigmented nail bands. When evaluating LM, a complete history should be obtained, including a detailed account of the pigmented nail band, in addition to medications and social and family histories. The physical examination should include all the digits and nail units and be accompanied by quality photography. The ABCDEF rule incorporates key components from the history and clinical examination and is helpful when evaluating LM. Histopathology remains the gold standard for diagnosis of LM if subungual melanoma is suspected.

Epidemiology

Subungual melanoma is a relatively rare neoplasm, with a reported incidence of 0.7–3.5% among all melanomas in the general population (Quinn et al. 1996; Finley et al. 1994). LM is a common presenting sign in a patient with nail apparatus melanoma, but only two of three patients with early-stage nail melanoma seek medical attention, often leading to a delay in diagnosis and a worse prognosis than cutaneous melanoma (Mendonça et al. 2004; Duarte et al. 2010). Subungual melanoma is more common among African--American, Native American, and Asian patients, with no gender preference, and the peak incidence is between the fifth and seventh decades (Mendonça et al. 2004; Koga et al. 2011; Braun et al. 2007).

History of the Diagnosis of Subungual Melanoma

Subungual melanoma was first described in 1834 by Boyer (1834) and by Hutchinson in 1886. Before 2000, diagnosis of nail unit melanoma was based on history and a clinical examination of the nail. In 2000, the ABCDEF rule was introduced to increase public and physician awareness and thus aid in the early detection of subungual melanoma (Levit et al. 2000). In 2001, publications began documenting the use of dermoscopy as a tool to help evaluate LM (Johr and Izakovic 2001; Ronger et al. 2002). Histopathology remains the gold standard for diagnosing subungual melanoma.

Differential Diagnosis

Exogenous pigment may be deposited onto the nail plate and examples include dirt, tobacco, potassium permanganate, and tar. These substances are usually easily differentiated from melanin because they do not form a vertical band. Most exogenous staining can be removed with scraping. Application of 5–10% ascorbic acid reduces permanganate to a colorless compound. Silver nitrate, which is used in the cauterization of granulation tissue, may show irregular staining of the nail plate and an adjacent discoloration of the nail folds. In cases of exogenous pigmentation, histopathology may neither show these substances nor uncover evidence of melanin (Haneke and Baran 2001).

Gram-negative bacteria, such as *Pseudomonas aeruginosa*, produce a greenish color on the nail plate and *Klebsiella*, and *Proteus* spp., give rise to gray–black pigment. This pigmentation can be differentiated from melanin by its characteristic origin at the junction of the proximal and lateral nail folds or the lateral nail groove with subsequent spreading over the rest of the nail plate, with irregularity of the medial border. Bacterial culture and/or histopathology are also helpful in elucidating the etiology (Haneke and Baran 2001).

Dermatophytes and nondermatophytes may produce a soluble, nongranular melanin with resulting brown to black discoloration of the nail plate. Fungal melanin can be differentiated from melanocytic melanin by the observation that dermatophyte pigmentation is typically wider distally at the hyponychium than proximally, and that the black band may have several jagged projections proximally. Histopathology shows both yellowish-brown pigmentation of the nail along with fungal hyphae in the subungual keratotic debris. The melanin can be seen within the hyphae and/or spores. Nondermatophytes such as *Scytalidium dimidiatum*, *Aspergillus niger*, *Exophiala*, *Wangiella* spp., and *Alternaria alternata* commonly cause a more diffuse brown nail pigmentation (Haneke and Baran 2001).

Blood is the leading cause of dark pigmentation of the nail and in most cases, it can be easily distinguished from malignancy. A subungual hematoma resulting from significant trauma is frequently clearly recollected by the patient because of the associated pain. Typically, there is leukonychia overlying the hematoma and the blood does not reach the free margin of the nail. Figure 3.1 shows a subungual hematoma of the hallux after the patient sustained an acute trauma. In addition to the brown-violaceous pigment involving most of the nail plate, there is a transverse fissure with partial detachment of the nail plate, corresponding to the point of impact. A hematoma from repeated minimal trauma, such as that from tight-fitting shoes may present as a vertical ellipse rather than a longitudinal band. Serial photography can aid diagnosis as can the application of a drop of immersion oil on the nail plate in conjunction with a strong magnifier lens or dermatoscope, revealing tiny globules of dried blood. It should be noted that the presence of blood may camouflage a nail melanoma. If suspicion persists, a punch biopsy of the nail plate should be sent for histopathology (Haneke and Baran 2001).

Melanocytes are normally present in the nail matrix, but in much lower amounts than found in normal skin. Ten percent of melanocytes are located in the proximal matrix, whereas 90% are in the distal matrix (Di Chiacchio et al. 2013). There are even fewer nail bed melanocytes than in the nail matrix and they do not synthesize melanin (Perrin et al. 1997; Tosti et al. 1994). This finding explains why nail bed melanomas are often amelanotic (Di Chiacchio et al. 2013). Nail matrix melanocytes may be active in darker skinned individuals, especially in adults, but they are

Fig. 3.1 Subungual hematoma of the hallux following acute trauma

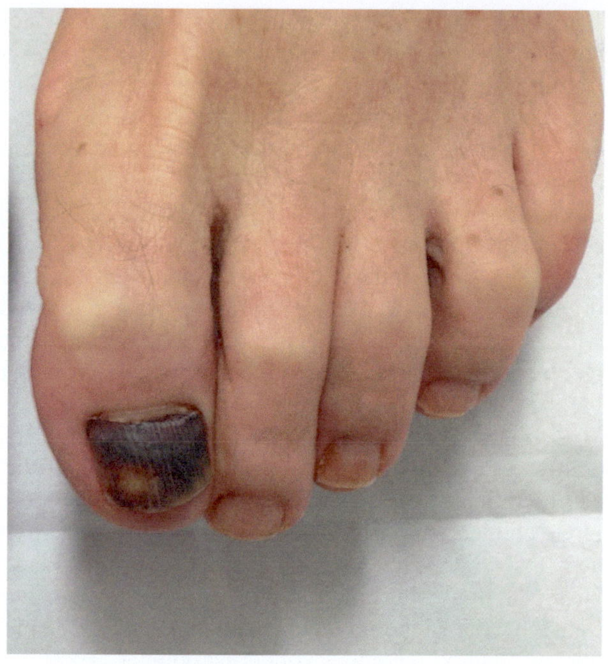

typically quiescent in Caucasians. A longitudinal brown to black band appears when melanocytes are activated and produce melanin in excess quantities that cannot be degraded by matrix keratinocytes (Haneke and Baran 2001; Braun et al. 2007; Andre and Lateur 2006). LM may be the result of benign processes such as benign melanocytic activation, lentigines and nevi, or malignant conditions such as melanoma (Zaiac 2002).

Benign melanocytic activation is characterized by increased melanocytic activity, but no increase in melanocyte number, resulting in a circumscribed pigmented macule in the matrix (Tosti et al. 1994). The melanocytes are typically dendritic and there may be some scattered melanophages (Ruben 2010). Some etiologies include trauma and friction (Baran 1987). Medications may also cause activation of nail matrix melanocytes and although the mechanism is not well understood, data suggest that it might be independent of melanocyte-stimulating hormone (MSH), adrenocorticotropic hormone (ACTH) activity, and ultraviolet light. Some examples of drugs causing pigmented nail bands are azathioprine, zidovudine, psoralens, and chemotherapeutic agents. Even when a causative drug is identified and discontinued, LM may persist for months to years (Baran and Kechijian 1989; Piraccini et al. 2006), which is often frustrating for both physicians and patients.

Lentigo simplex is characterized by a slight or moderate increase in matrical melanocytes (Amin et al. 2008). Dendritic melanocytes and a limited number of melanophages may also be observed (Ruben 2010). Melanocytic nevi are similar to lentigines; however, nests are also present. Most nevi of the nail apparatus are junctional, and there may be associated periungual pigmentation, which is more common in the pediatric population (Tosti et al. 1996; Leaute-Labreze et al. 1996; Goettmann-Bonvallot et al. 1999).

An increased number of melanocytes with larger hyperchromatic, pleomorphic nuclei and prominent nucleoli characterize atypical melanocytic hyperplasia (Di Chiacchio et al. 2013). Malignant melanoma in situ is difficult to diagnose histologically, even by highly trained dermatopathologists (Di Chiacchio et al. 2013). Important criteria that are used to diagnose nail unit melanoma include more frequent mitoses and long branching dendrites (Kopf and Waldo 1980), poor circumscription, increased density of intraepidermal melanocytes, irregular distribution of melanocytes with a confluence of nests, and cytological atypia (Di Chiacchio et al. 2013). Most subungual melanomas are of the acrolentiginous type (Clark et al. 1979).

Fortunately, benign melanocytic activation and nevi are the most common causes of LM in adults and children respectively (Ruben 2010; Andre and Lateur 2006). The diagnosis of LM is based on a combination of clinical history, worrisome clinical features, and the ABCDEF rule (Levit et al. 2000). Dermoscopy may also be a helpful tool (discussed in Chaps. 5 and 6), but histological examination is the final word in diagnosis (Adigun and Scher 2012). Although nail melanomas are less common than benign conditions, awareness of melanoma-associated LM reduces the likelihood of delayed diagnosis and improves patient outcomes (Cohen et al. 2008). In fact, most linear pigmentations that are not benign show melanoma in situ histologically. Notably, as opposed to cutaneous melanoma, in which 80% of cases are diagnosed at the TNM (tumor size and/or extent, regional lymph node involvement, metastases) stage I, only 20% of subungual melanomas are diagnosed at this early stage. Over 50% of patients with subungual melanoma die |within 5 years of diagnosis (Mendonça et al. 2004).

Patient History

A thorough history is critical in the initial consultation for LM and an interval history should be obtained at subsequent visits. Table 3.1 summarizes elements of the history that are concerning with regard to a subungual melanoma.

Age is important in the evaluation of nail melanoma because the age of presentation ranges from 20 to 90 years, with few cases presenting in infants and children (Levit et al. 2000). Although the peak incidence of nail melanoma is between the fifth and seventh decades of life, a full nail examination should be performed on patients of all ages, as malignancy can present at any age (Iorizzo et al. 2008).

The patient should be asked about LM onset and duration in addition to changes, such as color, width of the band, bleeding, or changes in the quality of the nail plate. Specifically, rapid growth and changes in shape and color may be concerning with regard to subungual melanoma.

Race is another diagnostic consideration, with African–Americans, Native Americans, and Asians over-represented in cases of subungual melanoma (Levit et al. 2000). Notably, although subungual melanoma is more common in darker

Table 3.1 Important elements of the history in the evaluation of longitudinal melanonychia (LM)

Feature	More likely subungual melanoma	Less likely subungual melanoma
Age	5th–7th decades	Infants, children
Race	African–Americans, Native Americans and Asians	Caucasians
Medications	No previous medications or medication with no association with LM	Previous or current use of bleomycin, fluoride, melphalan, cyclophosphamide, doxorubicin, paclitaxel, antimalarials, zidovudine, azathioprine, psoralens, quinacrine, doxorubicin, cyclophosphamide, nitrogen mustard, methotrexate, blood thinners (i.e., aspirin)
Onset/duration of pigmented nail band	Sudden appearance	Stable over many years or present since childhood
Change in pigmented nail band (color, width, shape of band)	Yes	No
Other diseases and conditions	No systemic diseases or conditions	Addison's disease, following bilateral adrenalectomy for Cushing's disease, scleroderma, leprosy, Laugier–Hunziker syndrome, lichen planus
Social history	Sedentary lifestyle, desk job, frequent wearing of flip flops or sneakers, trauma or bleeding[a]	Sports, exercise, trauma, employment involving physical labor or extended periods of standing, tight fitting shoes, high-heeled shoes
Personal and/or family history of cutaneous melanoma and/or atypical nevi	Present	None
History of application of exogenous pigment (dirt, tobacco, potassium permanganate, tar, silver nitrate)	No	Yes
History or evidence of bacterial or fungal nail infection	No	Yes

[a]Note that a history of trauma of bleeding may be associated with subungual melanoma

skinned patients, for reasons not entirely understood, the incidence of cutaneous melanoma is less common in subjects with colored skin than in lighter skinned individuals. Subungual melanoma accounts for 15–20% of all melanomas in African–Americans (Baran and Kechijian 1989), 10–31% in Asians (Finley et al. 1994; Baran and Kechijian 1989; Kato et al. 1996; Saida 1989; Takematsu et al. 1985), and 33% in Native Americans (Black and Wiggins 1985).

Medications may cause longitudinal pigmentation of the nail; thus, a list of current and past drugs, in addition to start and stop dates, should be obtained.

Some medications known to cause LM are bleomycin, fluoride, melphalan, cyclophosphamide, doxorubicin, paclitaxel, antimalarials, zidovudine, azathioprine, and psoralens. Dark transverse bands may also be associated with quinacrine, doxorubicin, and cyclophosphamide. Nitrogen mustard and methotrexate may produce diffuse hyperpigmentation of the nail plate (Lipner and Scher 2016).

A thorough history of systemic diseases and dermatological conditions should also be recorded. Longitudinal pigmented bands associated with systemic disorders are usually present in multiple nails, and have been reported in Addison's disease, following bilateral adrenalectomy for Cushing's disease, in scleroderma, and in leprosy (Lipner and Scher 2016). Laugier–Hunziker syndrome is a rare acquired disorder characterized by diffuse gray to dark brown macules, predominantly on the lips and oral mucosa, without systemic manifestations. About 50% of patients also have accompanying longitudinal melanonychia of their fingernails (Makhoul et al. 2003). Typical features characterize lichen planus of the nails, such as longitudinal ridging, nail plate thinning, and pterygium, and there may be associated LM (Baran et al. 1985; Juhlin and Baran 1989). Figure 3.2 shows a patient with longstanding nail lichen planus with nail plate dystrophy and atrophy along with LM involving multiple nails.

A social history including sports activities, such as soccer or long distance running, with repetitive contact of the nail with footwear, may raise the suspicion of subungual hematoma. Patients should also be asked about their occupations, specifically whether they have an active profession or a desk job. Patients who do manual labor or very physical jobs with long periods of standing and walking many be more prone to trauma. The physician should ask about acute trauma to the hands or feet, such as a history of dropping an object on their toe, stubbing their toe, or a digit being caught in a door. In addition, blood thinners, such as aspirin, may facilitate subungual hemorrhage when there is accompanying trauma (Braun et al. 2007). A history of trauma is also frequently reported in patients with subungual melanoma, but the pathogenesis is not understood (Tan et al. 2007).

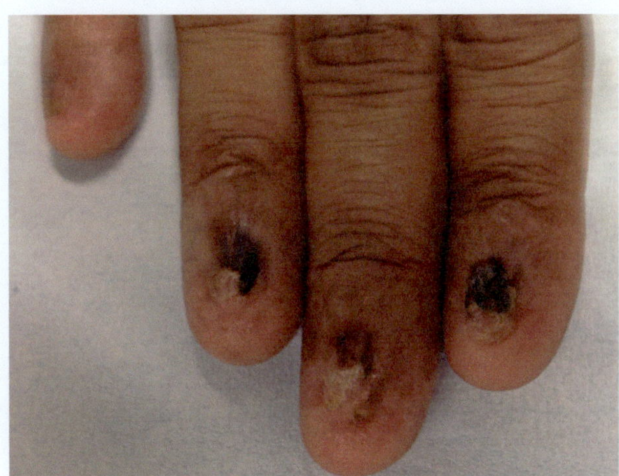

Fig. 3.2 Nail lichen planus with nail plate dystrophy, atrophy, and longitudinal melanonychia

Finally, personal and family histories of cutaneous melanoma and atypical nevi should be elicited because these characteristics all raise the suspicion of a subungual melanoma or future malignant degeneration of nail melanotic macules (Baran and Kechijian 1989; Kelly et al. 1997).

Clinical Examination

A detailed examination of LM is essential because certain clinical findings are more common with subungual melanomas in contrast to benign conditions. Serial photography should be standard practice to document changes over time. Neither a reliable patient nor an impeccable medical record can substitute for the detail and resolution afforded by quality images. Important elements of the physical examination include which and how many digits are affected, hand dominance, color(s) of the band, pigment homogeneity, band width, band borders, the presence or absence of pigment on the surrounding skin and any associated nail dystrophy, ulceration or blood (Haneke and Baran 2001; Andre and Lateur 2006). Table 3.2 summarizes signs that may be concerning for subungual melanoma.

The likelihood of malignancy is higher when a pigmented band involves a single digit as opposed to bands noted on many digits (Baran and Kechijian 1989; Glat et al. 1996; Shukla and Hughes 1989; Beltrani and Scher 1991). Multiple nails with LM are much more common in dark-skinned individuals. Of note, nearly 100% of patients with darker skin types exhibit LM by age 50 (Andre and Lateur 2006). Nevertheless, in patients with LM affecting more than one nail, each band should be examined, followed over time, and the physician must have a low threshold for biopsy if one or more of these bands exhibits concerning changes.

Nail melanoma may occur in any digit, but it is most common in the thumb, hallux, and index finger respectively (Haneke and Baran 2001; Andre and Lateur 2006;

Table 3.2 Important clinical signs in the evaluation of LM

Clinical sign	More concerning with regard to subungual melanoma	Less concerning with regard to subungual melanoma
Number of digits	One	Multiple
Digit involved	Thumb, hallux, and index finger	Other digits
Hand dominance[a]	Dominant hand	Non-dominant hand
Band color	Heterogeneous brown and black, homogeneous black color or darker color	Homogeneous brown color or lighter color
Band border	Indistinct, blurred	Distinct, sharp
Band width	Greater than 6 mm	Less than 6 mm
Change in band	Expansion of pigmented band, change in color, change in nail morphology	No changes
Hutchinson's sign	Present	Absent or pseudo-Hutchinson's sign
Nail plate morphology	Splitting, fissuring, ulceration, blood	Normal

[a]Controversial

Husain et al. 2006). One study found that in cases of melanoma involving the hand, the dominant hand is more common (Glat et al. 1996), but another study did not confirm this finding (Quinn et al. 1996).

On clinical examination of LM, pigmented nail band typically appears brown or black (Molina and Sanchez 1995). There is a higher index of suspicion for melanoma when there is heterogeneous brown and black color or homogeneous black pigmentation, as opposed to benign conditions, which have homogenous brown color (Saida 1989). The nail band border should also be examined, with indistinct or blurred border more commonly seen with nail melanomas (Baran and Kechijian 1989; Saida 1989; Takematsu et al. 1985; Beltrani and Scher 1991; Scher and Silvers 1991). Figure 3.3 shows an example of benign nevi in two African–American patients. The band is a light brown color with sharp borders.

The width of the band is also an important factor with authors citing a breadth of 3 mm or more (Kato et al. 1989; Ackerman 1982), exceeding 5 mm (Ruben 2010), or greater than 6 mm (Mannava et al. 2013), as being concerning for subungual melanoma.

Other worrisome signs for melanoma are the sudden appearance of a band in a previous normal nail plate, expansion in the width of the pigmented band, and change in color (i.e., becoming homogenous black or heterogeneous brown–black) (Quinn et al. 1996; Baran and Kechijian 1989; Glat et al. 1996; Shukla and Hughes

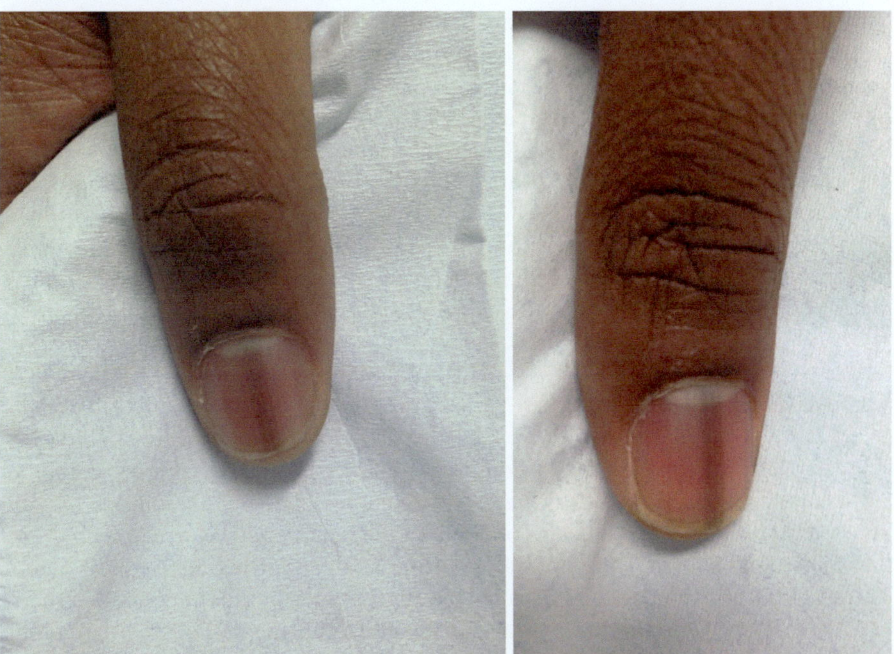

Fig. 3.3 Benign nevi in two African–American patients. The band is *light brown* with sharply defined borders

1989; Kato et al. 1989; Bibbo et al. 1994; Papachristou and Fortner 1982). A band that is wider proximally than distally (triangular shape) may be indicative of a growing neoplasm in an adult (Ruben 2010).

Another concerning finding is the extension of brown–black pigment from the nail bed, matrix, and nail plate onto the cuticle and lateral and/or proximal nail folds, known as Hutchinson's sign. It has been described as a complete or partial circle, a large spot, dash, or rod. Hutchinson's sign represents the clinical equivalent of the radial growth phase of subungual melanoma (Takematsu et al. 1985; Gibson 1957; Patterson and Helwig 1980). In addition, extension of the pigment onto the free edge of the nail plate is another sign that raises the suspicion of subungual melanoma (Baran and Kechijian 1996).

Although the presence of Hutchinson's sign may be worrisome for melanoma, there are a few caveats to keep in mind when evaluating LM. There are benign conditions with LM accompanied by periungual pigmentation, and in these cases the skin discoloration is known as pseudo-Hutchinson's sign (Baran and Kechijian 1996). Pseudo-Hutchinson's sign can be seen in Laugier–Hunziker syndrome (Baran and Kechijian 1989; Baran and Barriere 1986). Peutz–Jeghers syndrome (Baran and Kechijian 1989), normally in some African–American individuals (Baran and Kechijian 1996), following treatment with radiation to the digits (Shelley et al. 1964), trauma (Baran 1987), malnutrition (Bisht and Singh 1962), minocycline (Mooney and Bennett 1988), zidovudine (Baran and Kechijian 1989), in patients with AIDS (Gallais et al. 1992), a congenital nevus (Asahina et al. 1993), and following a nail unit biopsy (Kopf and Waldo 1980).

Other signs that may be indicative of nail melanoma are changes in nail plate morphology including dystrophy, such as nail fissuring or splitting, ulceration or blood under the nail plate (Mannava et al. 2013). Demonstration of subungual hematoma does not rule out a diagnosis of melanoma, because developing neoplasms may bleed (Haneke and Baran 2001; Andre and Lateur 2006; Daniel and Jellinek 2007).

While these features may be helpful in distinguishing between benign and malignant causes of LM, clinical examination alone may not be sufficient for a definitive diagnosis, necessitating a biopsy if suspicion persists.

The ABCDEF Rule

The ABCDEF rule for the evaluation of LM was first proposed as a mnemonic in 2000 and is routinely used in clinical practice today (Levit et al. 2000). This rule incorporates many of the key components of the history and clinical examination that have been shown to be important in the analysis of pigmented nail bands. The stimulus to formulate an LM rule stemmed from a similar mnemonic already used successfully in clinical practice to diagnose cutaneous melanomas, along with the high mortality, lack of public and physician awareness, late presentations, and misdiagnoses of subungual melanomas. For example, when subungual melanoma is finally diagnosed, about 15% of these tumors are already metastatic

(Pomerance et al. 1994). Notably, the mnemonic for cutaneous melanomas resulted in 80% of these malignancies being diagnosed at stage I (TNM classification) with a 5-year survival rate of up to 100% reported in some studies (Glat et al. 1996). The rule for skin melanomas was first presented in 1985 as the ABCD rule (Friedman et al. 1985), and then modified in 2004 to the ABCDE rule (Abbasi et al. 2004). It is important to be aware that while the mnemonics for cutaneous and subungual melanomas sound similar, they were invented by entirely different authors and have completely different meanings. A comparison of the ABCDE rule for cutaneous melanomas and the ABCDEF rule for subungual melanomas is summarized in Table 3.3.

In this system, the "A" signifies the *a*ge of presentation, namely the fifth to seventh decades, representing the peak incidence of subungual melanoma. The "A" also stands for the most commonly affected races: *A*frican-American, *N*ative *A*merican, and *A*sian (Levit et al. 2000).

The "B" in this system represents the pigmented nail *b*and, which is typically *b*rown or *b*lack. The "B" also stands for *b*readth/width (3 mm or more), and *b*order (irregular or *b*lurred) (Levit et al. 2000).

The letter "C" represents *c*hange in the pigmented band. Melanoma is more likely when there is a new, sudden, or rapid growth in the band, pigment variegation or change in nail morphology. Figure 3.4 shows an example of melanoma in situ, with heterogeneous brown and black pigmentation. Other worrisome signs are persistent or worsening nail plate dystrophy or ulceration. It should be noted that color changes are often absent in cases of amelanotic melanoma (Levit et al. 2000).

The "D" in this system stands for the *d*igit involved. The thumbs, followed by the hallux or index finger are the digits most frequently affected by subungual melanoma. The "D" also represents *d*ominance and single *d*igit, as malignancy is more

Table 3.3 Summary of the ABCDE rule for cutaneous melanoma and the ABCDEF rule for subungual melanomas (modified from (Levit et al. 2000; Abbasi et al. 2004))

Letter	Cutaneous melanoma	Subungual melanoma
A	Asymmetry	*A*ge: peak 5th–7th decades
		Race: *A*frican–American, *N*ative *A*merican, and *A*sian
B	Border irregularity	Pigmented nail *b*and: *b*rown or *b*lack
		*B*readth/width (3 mm or more)
		*B*order (irregular or *b*lurred)
C	Color variation	*C*hange in pigmented band: new, sudden, or rapid growth
		No *c*hange: no improvement in nail plate dystrophy or ulceration
D	Diameter greater than 6 mm	*D*igit affected: thumb, hallux, index finger
		Single *d*igit affected
		*D*ominant hand
E	Evolving (new or changing lesion)	*E*xtension of brown or black pigment to the proximal or lateral nail folds (Hutchinson's sign) or spreading of the pigment onto the free edge of the nail plate
F		*F*amily or personal history: cutaneous or subungual melanoma or atypical nevi

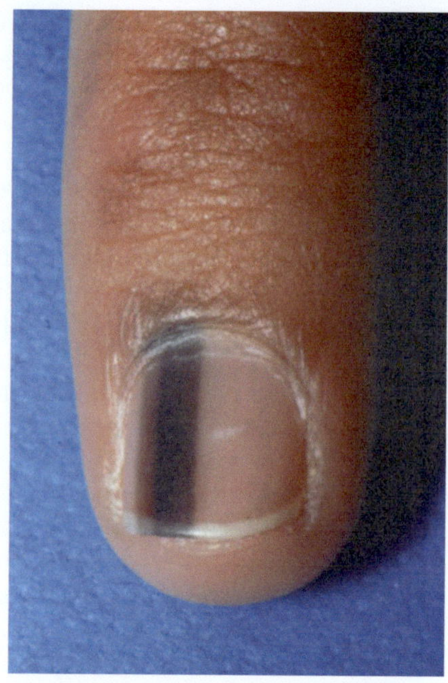

Fig. 3.4 Melanoma in situ, the band is heterogeneous with *brown* and *black* pigmentation

common when the band involves the dominant hand or a single digit, as opposed to multiple digits (Levit et al. 2000).

The "E" represents *e*xtension of the brown or black pigment to the proximal or lateral nail folds, also known as Hutchinson's sign, and spreading of the pigment onto the free edge of the nail plate, both of which raise the suspicion of subungual melanoma (Levit et al. 2000).

"F" is the last letter in this system, and represents *f*amily and/or personal history of dysplastic nevus syndrome or previous melanomas, both of which raise the suspicion of a subungual melanoma (Levit et al. 2000).

It is not required for LM to have all the ABCDEF features to suggest a diagnosis of melanoma. Rather, the index of suspicion is additive and supported by these features; LM meeting more criteria is more suggestive of subungual melanoma.

Limitations of the Clinical Evaluation of LM

In a report of 12 cases of melanonychias (5 melanomas and 7 nonmelanomas) analyzed by group of dermatologists with different levels of experience, the authors demonstrated the shortcomings of both clinical and dermoscopic evaluation of LM (Di Chiacchio et al. 2010). Of these 152 dermatologists, 11 were nail specialists, 53 were senior dermatologists (more than 10 years in practice), and 88 were junior dermatologists (less than 10 years in practice). Each clinician was asked to diagnose the LM cases based on four successive steps: clinical examination, evaluation utilizing the ABCDEF rule, dermoscopy of the nail plate, and intraoperative dermoscopy of the nail matrix. Of these four evaluations, the only method that statistically influenced the correct diagnosis was intraoperative dermoscopy. The overall accuracy of the group in the diagnosis of subungual melanoma was low, as the percentage of dermatologists stating the correct diagnosis using the first three methods ranged from just 46% to 55%. It was also concerning that nail plate dermoscopy did not improve the diagnostic accuracy, even amongst those dermatologists who were highly trained in the technique and identified themselves as experts in nail disorders (Di Chiacchio et al. 2010). This study highlights the limitations of clinical examination and utilizing the ABCDEF rule in the diagnosis of LM, and emphasizes the need for more research in this area and importance of histology.

Pediatric LM

Caution and modifications must be employed in utilizing the key concerning clinical features that apply to adult LM and applying the ABCDEF rule to the evaluation of LM in the pediatric population. As opposed to adults, in children, approximately 75% of pigmented bands can be attributed to melanocytic hyperplasia, predominately nevi, and the other 25% are the result of melanocyte activation (Richert and Andre 2011). Nevi originating in the nail matrix may be congenital or acquired, and usually affect the fingers, typically the thumb. Figure 3.5 shows an example of a benign nevus of the hallux in a 3-year-old girl. The band is triangular, i.e., wider at the proximal end than at the distal end. This feature would be concerning in an adult, but may represent a benign growing nevus in the pediatric population. Over 50% of childhood LM cases are greater than 3 mm wide, and periungual pigmentation may be present in up to a third of cases (Goettmann-Bonvallot et al. 1999; Richert and Andre 2011). The diagnosis of subungual melanoma is reported, but rarely in children, although it must be considered in the differential diagnosis of LM in a pediatric patient (Tosti et al. 2012; Antonovich et al. 2005).

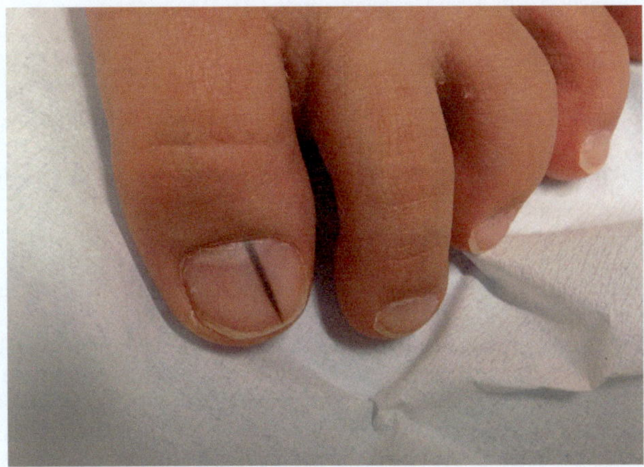

Fig. 3.5 Benign nevus of the hallux in a 3-year-old girl with a *triangular* band

Summary for the Physician

Malignant melanoma of the nail unit presents with a higher mortality rate than cutaneous melanoma, which is partially attributed to a poor prognosis due to delays in diagnosis. As approximately two-thirds of nail melanomas present clinically as LM, it is important that the physician understands how to properly evaluate pigmented nail bands. A thorough history and clinical examination of the nail unit is essential for early diagnosis of subungual melanomas. The ABCDEF rule is also helpful as a mnemonic to remember the key features indicating suspected malignancy. Histopathology remains the gold standard for the diagnosis of nail unit melanomas.

References

Abbasi NR, Shaw HM, Rigel DS, Friedman RJ, McCarthy WH, Osman I, et al. Early diagnosis of cutaneous melanoma: revisiting the ABCD criteria. JAMA. 2004;292(22):2771–6.

Ackerman AB. Conventional microscopy: signs that stamp pigmented melanocytic nevi as benign. Am J Dermatopathol. 1982;4(5):461–6.

Adigun CG, Scher RK. Longitudinal melanonychia: when to biopsy and is dermoscopy helpful? Dermatol Ther. 2012;25(6):491–7.

Amin B, Nehal KS, Jungbluth AA, Zaidi B, Brady MS, Coit DC, et al. Histologic distinction between subungual lentigo and melanoma. Am J Surg Pathol. 2008;32(6):835–43.

Andre J, Lateur N. Pigmented nail disorders. Dermatol Clin. 2006;24(3):329–39.

Antonovich DD, Grin C, Grant-Kels JM. Childhood subungual melanoma in situ in diffuse nail melanosis beginning as expanding longitudinal melanonychia. Pediatr Dermatol. 2005;22(3):210–2.

Asahina A, Chi HI, Otsuka F. Subungual pigmented nevus: evaluation of DNA ploidy in six cases. J Dermatol. 1993;20(8):466–72.

Baran R. Frictional longitudinal melanonychia: a new entity. Dermatologica. 1987;174(6):280–4.

Baran R, Barriere H. Longitudinal melanonychia with spreading pigmentation in Laugier-Hunziker syndrome: a report of two cases. Br J Dermatol. 1986;115(6):707–10.

Baran R, Kechijian P. Longitudinal melanonychia (melanonychia striata): diagnosis and management. J Am Acad Dermatol. 1989;21(6):1165–75.

Baran R, Kechijian P. Hutchinson's sign: a reappraisal. J Am Acad Dermatol. 1996;34(1):87–90.

Baran R, Jancovici E, Sayag J, Dawber RP. Longitudinal melanonychia in lichen planus. Br J Dermatol. 1985;113(3):369–70.

Beltrani VP, Scher RK. Evaluation and management of melanonychia striata in a patient receiving phototherapy. Arch Dermatol. 1991;127(3):319–20.

Bibbo C, Brolin RE, Warren AM, Franklin ID. Current therapy for subungual melanoma. J Foot Ankle Surg: Off Publ Am Coll Foot Ankle Surg. 1994;33(2):184–93.

Bisht DB, Singh SS. Pigmented bands on nails: a new sign in malnutrition. Lancet. 1962;1(7228):507–8.

Black WC, Wiggins C. Melanoma among southwestern American Indians. Cancer. 1985;55(12):2899–902.

Boyer A. Fungus hematide du petit doigt. Gaz Med Paris. 1834;212(13):212.

Braun RP, Baran R, Le Gal FA, Dalle S, Ronger S, Pandolfi R, et al. Diagnosis and management of nail pigmentations. J Am Acad Dermatol. 2007;56(5):835–47.

Clark WH, Bernardino E, Reed RJ, Kopf AW. Acral lentiginous melanomas. In: Clark WHGL, Mastrangero MJ, editors. Human malignant melanoma. New York: Stratton; 1979. p. 109–24.

Cohen T, Busam KJ, Patel A, Brady MS. Subungual melanoma: management considerations. Am J Surg. 2008;195(2):244–8.

Daniel 3rd CR, Jellinek NJ. Subungual blood is not always a reassuring sign. J Am Acad Dermatol. 2007;57(1):176.

Di Chiacchio N, Hirata SH, Enokihara MY, Michalany NS, Fabbrocini G, Tosti A. Dermatologists' accuracy in early diagnosis of melanoma of the nail matrix. Arch Dermatol. 2010;146(4):382–7.

Di Chiacchio N, Ruben BS, Loureiro WR. Longitudinal melanonychias. Clin Dermatol. 2013;31(5):594–601.

Duarte AF, Correia O, Barros AM, Azevedo R, Haneke E. Nail matrix melanoma in situ: conservative surgical management. Dermatology. 2010;220(2):173–5.

English C, Hammert WC. Cutaneous malignancies of the upper extremity. J Hand Surg. 2012;37(2):367–77.

Finley 3rd RK, Driscoll DL, Blumenson LE, Karakousis CP. Subungual melanoma: an eighteen-year review. Surgery. 1994;116(1):96–100.

Friedman RJ, Rigel DS, Kopf AW. Early detection of malignant melanoma: the role of physician examination and self-examination of the skin. CA Cancer J Clin. 1985;35(3):130–51.

Gallais V, Lacour JP, Perrin C, Ghanem G, Bodokh I, Ortonne JP. Acral hyperpigmented macules and longitudinal melanonychia in AIDS patients. Br J Dermatol. 1992;126(4):387–91.

Gibson SH, Montgomery H, Woolner B, Brunsting LA. Melanotic whitlow (subungual melanoma). J Invest Dermatol 1957;29:119–129.

Glat PM, Spector JA, Roses DF, Shapiro RA, Harris MN, Beasley RW, et al. The management of pigmented lesions of the nail bed. Ann Plast Surg. 1996;37(2):125–34.

Goettmann-Bonvallot S, Andre J, Belaich S. Longitudinal melanonychia in children: a clinical and histopathologic study of 40 cases. J Am Acad Dermatol. 1999;41(1):17–22.

Haneke E, Baran R. Longitudinal melanonychia. Dermatol Surg. 2001;27(6):580–4.

Husain S, Scher RK, Silvers DN, Ackerman AB. Melanotic macule of nail unit and its clinico-pathologic spectrum. J Am Acad Dermatol. 2006;54(4):664–7.

Hutchinson J. Melanosis often not black: melanotic whitlow. Br Med J. 1886;1:491.

Ilyas EN, Leinberry CF, Ilyas AM. Skin cancers of the hand and upper extremity. J Hand Surg. 2012;37(1):171–8.

Iorizzo M, Tosti A, Di Chiacchio N, Hirata SH, Misciali C, Michalany N, et al. Nail melanoma in children: differential diagnosis and management. Dermatol Surg. 2008;34(7):974–8.

Johr RH, Izakovic J. Dermatoscopy/ELM for the evaluation of nail-apparatus pigmentation. Dermatol Surg. 2001;27(3):315–22.

Juhlin L, Baran R. Longitudinal melanonychia after healing of lichen planus. Acta Derm Venereol. 1989;69(4):338–9.

Kato T, Usuba Y, Takematsu H, Kumasaka N, Tanita Y, Hashimoto K, et al. A rapidly growing pigmented nail streak resulting in diffuse melanosis of the nail. A possible sign of subungual melanoma in situ. Cancer. 1989;64(10):2191–7.

Kato T, Suetake T, Sugiyama Y, Tabata N, Tagami H. Epidemiology and prognosis of subungual melanoma in 34 Japanese patients. Br J Dermatol. 1996;134(3):383–7.

Kelly JW, Yeatman JM, Regalia C, Mason G, Henham AP. A high incidence of melanoma found in patients with multiple dysplastic naevi by photographic surveillance. Med J Aust. 1997;167(4):191–4.

Koga H, Saida T, Uhara H. Key point in dermoscopic differentiation between early nail apparatus melanoma and benign longitudinal melanonychia. J Dermatol. 2011;38(1):45–52.

Kopf AW, Waldo E. Melanonychia striata. Australas J Dermatol. 1980;21(2):59–70.

Leaute-Labreze C, Bioulac-Sage P, Taieb A. Longitudinal melanonychia in children. A study of eight cases. Arch Dermatol. 1996;132(2):167–9.

Levit EK, Kagen MH, Scher RK, Grossman M, Altman E. The ABC rule for clinical detection of subungual melanoma. J Am Acad Dermatol. 2000;42(2 Pt 1):269–74.

Lipner S, Scher, RK. Nail signs of systemic diseases. In: Callen J, Jorizzo, JL., editor. Dermatological signs of systemic disease. 5th ed. Amsterdam: Elsevier; 2016.

Makhoul EN, Ayoub NM, Helou JF, Abadjian GA. Familial Laugier-Hunziker syndrome. J Am Acad Dermatol. 2003;49(2 Suppl Case Reports):S143–5.

Mannava KA, Mannava S, Koman LA, Robinson-Bostom L, Jellinek N. Longitudinal melanonychia: detection and management of nail melanoma. Hand Surg: Int J Devoted Hand Upper Limb Surg Relat Res: J Asia Pac Fed Soc Surg Hand. 2013;18(1):133–9.

Mendonça IRSMKB, Silva RT, Spinelli LP, Orofino RR, França JR. Melanoma do aparelho ungueal. An Bras Dermatol. 2004;79:575–80.

Molina D, Sanchez JL. Pigmented longitudinal bands of the nail. A clinicopathologic study. Am J Dermatopathol. 1995;17(6):539–41.

Mooney E, Bennett RG. Periungual hyperpigmentation mimicking Hutchinson's sign associated with minocycline administration. J Dermatol Surg Oncol. 1988;14(9):1011–3.

Papachristou DN, Fortner JG. Melanoma arising under the nail. J Surg Oncol. 1982;21(4):219–22.

Patterson RH, Helwig EB. Subungual malignant melanoma: a clinical-pathologic study. Cancer. 1980;46(9):2074–87.

Perrin C, Michiels JF, Pisani A, Ortonne JP. Anatomic distribution of melanocytes in normal nail unit: an immunohistochemical investigation. Am J Dermatopathol. 1997;19(5):462–7.

Piraccini BM, Iorizzo M, Starace M, Tosti A. Drug-induced nail diseases. Dermatol Clin. 2006;24(3):387–91.

Pomerance J, Kopf AW, Ramos L, Waldo E, Grossman JA. A large, pigmented nail bed lesion in a child. Ann Plast Surg. 1994;33(1):80–2.

Quinn MJ, Thompson JE, Crotty K, McCarthy WH, Coates AS. Subungual melanoma of the hand. J Hand Surg. 1996;21(3):506–11.

Richert B, Andre J. Nail disorders in children: diagnosis and management. Am J Clin Dermatol. 2011;12(2):101–12.

Ronger S, Touzet S, Ligeron C, Balme B, Viallard AM, Barrut D, et al. Dermoscopic examination of nail pigmentation. Arch Dermatol. 2002;138(10):1327–33.

Ruben BS. Pigmented lesions of the nail unit: clinical and histopathologic features. Semin Cutan Med Surg. 2010;29(3):148–58.

Saida T, Ohshima Y. Clinical and histopathological characteristicsof the early lesions of subungual melanoma. Cancer. 1989;63:556–60.

Scher RK, Silvers DN. Longitudinal melanonychia striata. J Am Acad Dermatol. 1991;24(6 Pt 1):1035–6.

Shelley WB, Rawnsley HM, Pillsbury DM. Postirradiation melanonychia. Arch Dermatol. 1964;90:174–6.

Shukla VK, Hughes LE. Differential diagnosis of subungual melanoma from a surgical point of view. Br J Surg. 1989;76(11):1156–60.

Takematsu H, Obata M, Tomita Y, Kato T, Takahashi M, Abe R. Subungual melanoma. A clinicopathologic study of 16 Japanese cases. Cancer. 1985;55(11):2725–31.

Tan KB, Moncrieff M, Thompson JF, McCarthy SW, Shaw HM, Quinn MJ, et al. Subungual melanoma: a study of 124 cases highlighting features of early lesions, potential pitfalls in diagnosis, and guidelines for histologic reporting. Am J Surg Pathol. 2007;31(12):1902–12.

Tosti A, Cameli N, Piraccini BM, Fanti PA, Ortonne JP. Characterization of nail matrix melanocytes with anti-PEP1, anti-PEP8, TMH-1, and HMB-45 antibodies. J Am Acad Dermatol. 1994;31(2 Pt 1):193–6.

Tosti A, Baran R, Piraccini BM, Cameli N, Fanti PA. Nail matrix nevi: a clinical and histopathologic study of twenty-two patients. J Am Acad Dermatol. 1996;34(5 Pt 1):765–71.

Tosti A, Piraccini BM, Cagalli A, Haneke E. In situ melanoma of the nail unit in children: report of two cases in fair-skinned Caucasian children. Pediatr Dermatol. 2012;29(1):79–83.

Zaiac MN, Daniel CR. Nails in systemic disease. Dermatol Ther. 2002;15(2):99–106.

Dermoscopy of the Nail Plate, Nail Matrix, and Nail Bed

4

Nilton Di Chiacchio, Diego L. Bet, and Nilton Gioia Di Chiacchio

> **Key Features**
> - Dermoscopy of the nail unit allows better characterization of pigmented lesions compared with the naked eye.
> - Dermoscopy easily differentiates subungual hemorrhages from melanin inclusions, and may reveal clues regarding the diagnosis of fungal melanonychia.
> - Background and lines are evaluated on dermoscopy of the nail plate, according to the color and regularity of the pattern.
> - Gray usually indicates melanocytic activation, whereas brown indicates melanocytic hyperplasia. Sometimes it may be hard to differentiate gray from light brown.
> - An irregular brown/black pattern may indicate a melanoma of the nail unit. Intraoperative polarized dermoscopy of the nail matrix and nail bed allows direct visualization and better characterization of pigmented lesions originating longitudinal melanonychia.
> - Four main patterns are described and validated for dermoscopy of the nail matrix and bed:
>   1. *Gray regular pattern*: indicates melanocytic activation
>   2. *Regular brown lines*: indicate benign melanocytic hyperplasia

N. Di Chiacchio (✉) • D.L. Bet
Hospital do Servidor Público Municipal, São Paulo, Brazil

N.G. Di Chiacchio
Hospital do Servidor Público Municipal, São Paulo, Brazil

Medical School of ABC, São Paulo, Brazil

© Springer International Publishing Switzerland 2017
N. Di Chiacchio, A. Tosti (eds.), *Melanonychias*,
DOI 10.1007/978-3-319-44993-7_4

> 3. *Regular lines with regular globules and blotches*: indicate *lentigo and melanocytic nevis*
> 4. *Irregular pattern*: favors a melanoma of the nail matrix
> - These dermoscopic patterns demonstrate good histopathological correlation and enhance diagnosis accuracy, even for non–nail experts.
> - Intraoperative dermoscopy permits better characterization of surgical margins for biopsy and excision, aiding the surgical management of longitudinal melanonychias.

Dermoscopy of the Nail Plate

Diagnosis of longitudinal melanonychia (LM) is usually difficult and remains a challenge for dermatologists (Di Chiacchio et al. 2013a). Clinical features are not always sufficient to obtain the correct diagnosis; thus, some other tools were developed to help to distinguish benign and malignant lesions, and also to avoid unnecessary biopsies (Di Chiacchio et al. 2013b). Dermoscopy (dermatoscopy, epiluminescence microscopy) is a noninvasive diagnostic technique for the in vivo observation of pigmented skin lesions. Dermoscopy of the nail plate has been described since around 1994, but only a few observations have been published (Johr and Izakovic 2001; Kawabata et al. 2001; Marghoob et al. 2004).

Technique

Polarized and nonpolarized devices may be used for nail plate dermoscopy. There is no evidence for consensus on which instrument and which light source are the most effective. The color and definition of the lines may vary among the different devices, so it is advisable to use the same device in the follow-up evaluations. The recommended magnification is ×10 (standard in portable dermatoscopes) because it allows visualization of the whole nail plate in the lens field, and better evaluation of the regularity of lines (Di Chiacchio et al. 2013a). When immersion fluid is needed, the best is ultrasound gel, because its lower viscosity permits it to stay on the nail plate and fill any concavities without rolling off (Ronger et al. 2002).

Video dermatoscopes with magnifications up to ×200 may also be used, but the convexity and hardness of the nail plate make it difficult to obtain a complete apposition of the dermatoscope lens to the surface (Piraccini et al. 2015) (Fig. 4.1).

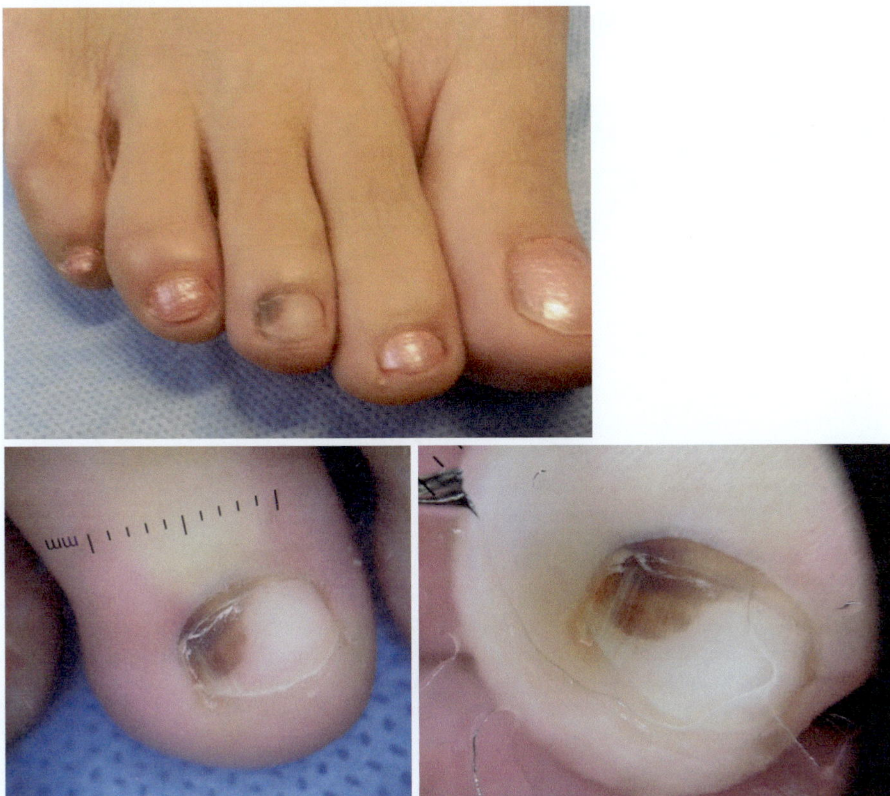

Fig. 4.1 Benefits of ultrasound gel for dermoscopy of the nail plate: on the *right*, fewer artifacts and better visualization of colors and lines (Pictures taken with the same dermatoscope and camera)

Dermoscopic Patterns Observed on the Nail Apparatus

Nail Plate Surface

Two important features need to be evaluated: background and lines. The background may be gray or brown, and lines as regular or irregular according to the regularity of coloration, spacing, thickness, and parallelism (Braun et al. 2007; Ronger et al. 2002).

A grayish background may vary from light to dark and is almost always associated with regular thin gray lines. This pattern is seen in cases of hypermelanosis resulting from melanocyte activation without melanocytic hyperplasia.

A brown background may also vary from light to dark, and the lines appearing with either a regular or an irregular pattern according to coloration, spacing, thickness, and parallelism. This pattern is associated with melanocytic hyperplasia.

Another pattern described and known as "blood spots" is characterized by well-circumscribed dots or blotches with purple–blue to brown coloration. This pattern almost never has a linear pattern, as observed in LM (Schema 4.1).

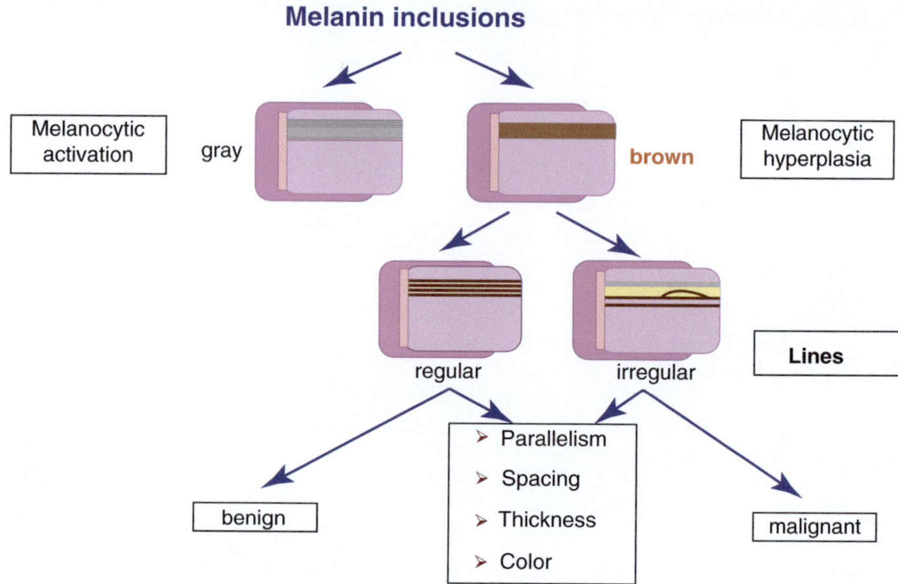

Schema 4.1 Algorithm for dermoscopy diagnosis of nail pigmentation. Grayish color is suggestive of focal melanocytic activation. Brownish color is suggestive for melanocytic hyperplasia. The lesions should be evaluated according to the pigmented lines. Regular lines suggest diagnosis of benign lesions, and irregular lines suggest the possibility of melanoma. (Adapted from Braun et al. (2007) and Ronger et al. (2002))

Free Edge of the Nail Plate

Examination of the free edge of the nail plate is useful for determining the origin of the pigmentation, and consequently which part of the matrix should be biopsied. When the pigment appears in the upper portion of the nail plate it means that the pigment was produced in the proximal nail matrix. On the other hand, if it appears in the lower part of the nail plate, it was produced in the distal matrix, which is the most common origin of LM (Braun et al. 2007).

Periungual Area

Pseudo-Hutchinson's Sign

It appears when the pigmentation is observed through the cuticle and the distal part of the nail folds due to its transparency. It commonly appears in nevi, but can also be observed in other conditions, such as Addison's disease, AIDS, Bowen's disease, drug administration, pigmentation, Laugier–Hunziker syndrome, malnutrition, Peutz–Jeghers syndrome, racial pigmentations (phototypes V and VI), radiation therapy, and trauma (Baran and Kechijian 1989; Lazaridou et al. 2013) (Fig. 4.2).

Micro-Hutchinson Sign

Micro-Hutchinson sign is defined as a pigmentation of the periungual area that can only be observed by dermoscopy examination and not with the naked eye (Ronger et al. 2002).

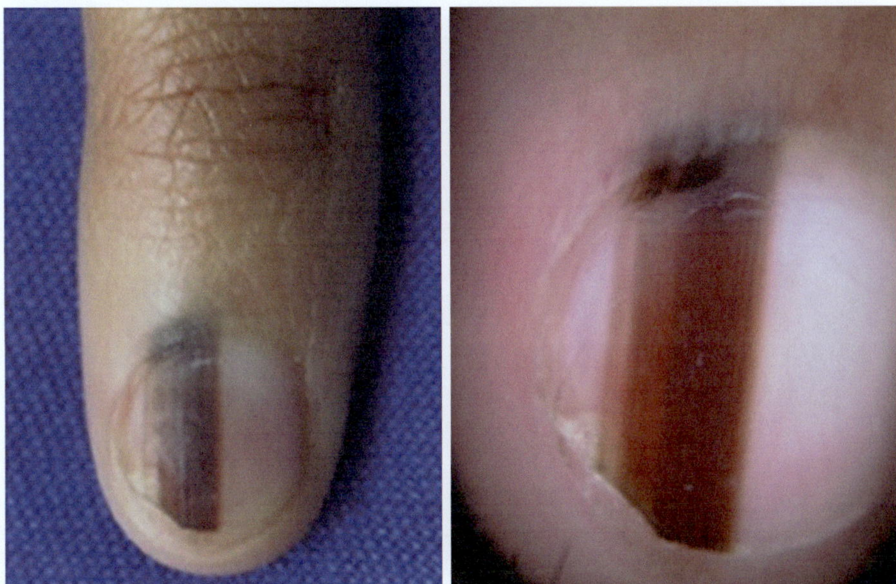

Fig. 4.2 Nevus with longitudinal melanonychia (LM) showing extension of the pigmentation to the periungual area suggestive of Hutchinson's sign. On dermoscopy, we see that the pigment is seen through the transparency of the cuticle and nail fold

Hutchinson's Sign

Hutchinson's sign is considered to be a periungual spread of pigmentation into the nail folds. Although it is a presumptive sign of nail melanoma, it has also been observed in nevi (Baran and Kechijian 1989).

Pigmentation with a brushed linear pattern across the skin marks was observed in nevi, whereas pigmentation distributed in a disorganized fashion over the entire surface was observed in melanomas (Kawabata et al. 2001).

Patterns Observed According to the Diagnosis of LM

Hypermelanosis

Clinically, hypermelanosis may be seen as horizontal or longitudinal stripes or as diffuse nail darkening. Under dermoscopic examination homogeneous grayish strips and gray lines are observed (Braun et al. 2007). Sometimes, it may be difficult to distinguish a light brown background from a gray background. Coloration may vary because of the Tyndall effect, depending on nail thickness and location of melanin within the nail plate (Di Chiacchio et al. 2013a) (Figs. 4.3, 4.4, and 4.5).

Lentigo

Dermoscopy shows parallel homogeneous grayish or brownish lines placed side by side, resulting in an appearance of a homogeneous gray or light brown pigmented strip. Melanin inclusions that identify it to be a lesion of melanocytic origin may also be observed (Ronger et al. 2002) (Fig. 4.6).

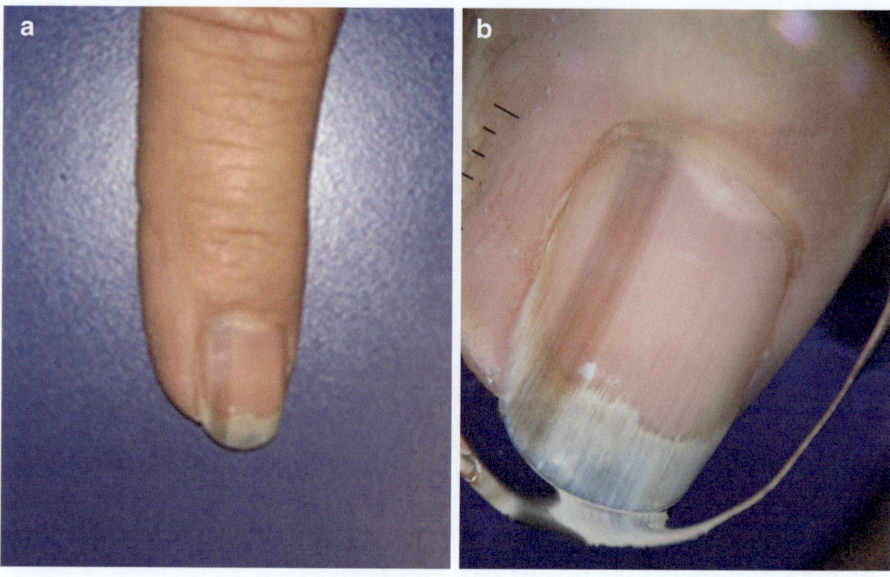

Fig. 4.3 (**a**) Fingernail with a longitudinal band with shades of *gray/brown*. (**b**) Dermoscopy of the nail plate: regular *gray* pattern, homogeneous *gray* background with barely visible lines

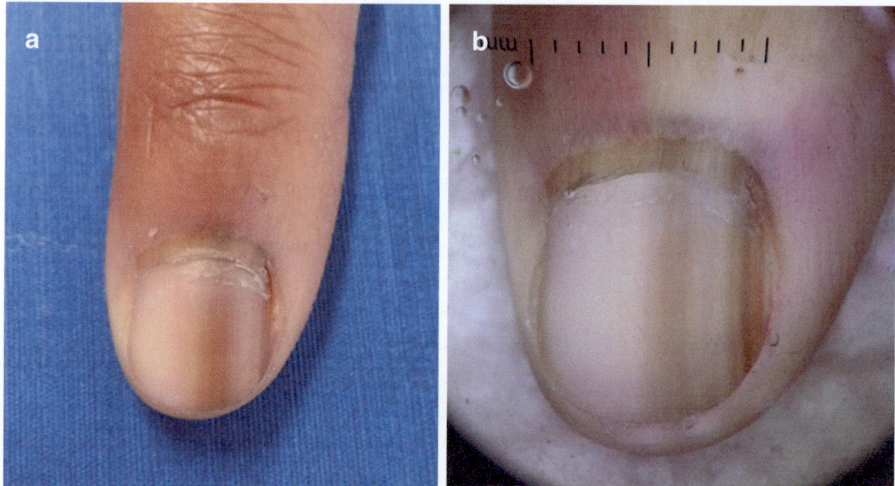

Fig. 4.4 (**a**) Fingernail with a longitudinal band with shades of *gray/brown*. (**b**) Dermoscopy of the nail plate: asymmetric band with a central structureless/homogeneous *gray* background varying in color intensity, lines varying in thickness and color, but maintaining regularity in spacing and color throughout its longitudinal growth

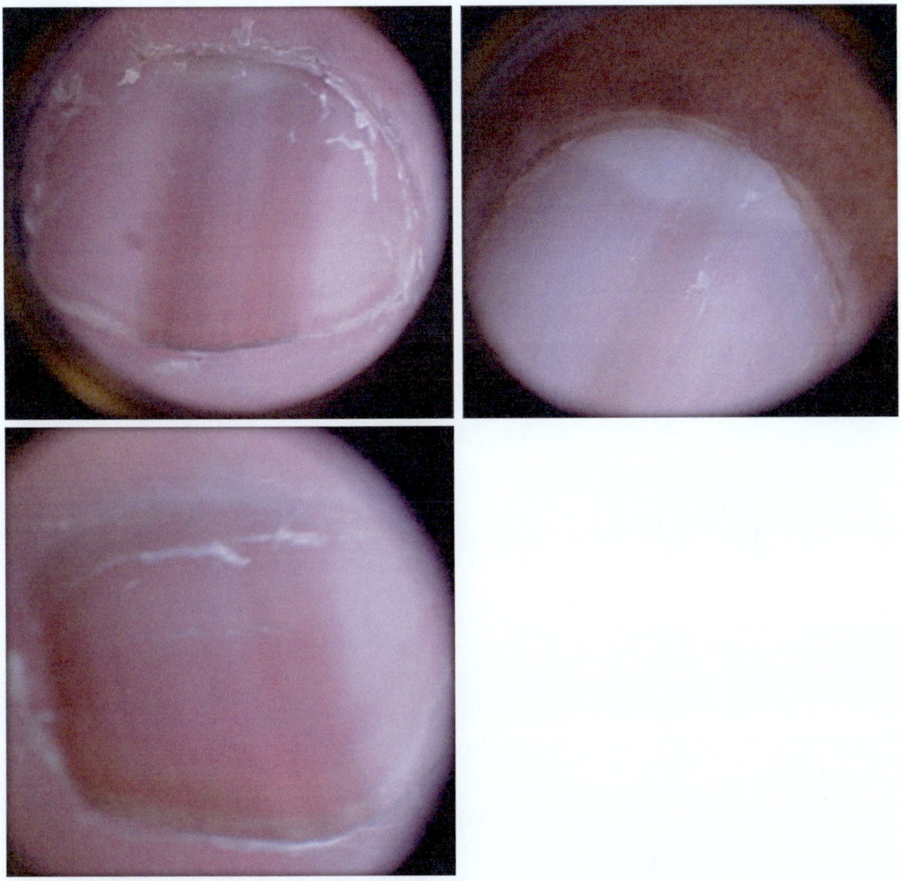

Fig. 4.5 Hypermelanosis: is it *gray* or *brown*? Sometimes it may be difficult to distinguish *light brown* from *gray*

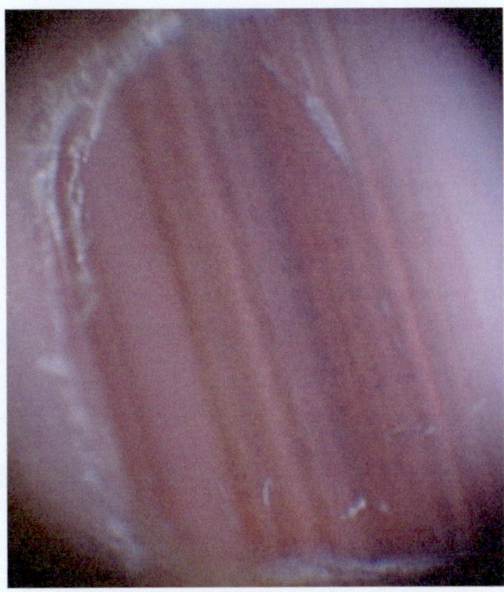

Fig. 4.6 Lentigo: regular *brown* and *gray* lined pattern on a light *gray* background

Nevi of the Nail Matrix

Dermoscopically, the global pattern observed in nevi of the nail matrix is considered to be regular, showing a homogeneous brown stripe with longitudinal parallel lines that have regular spacing and thickness (Ronger et al. 2002) (Figs. 4.7, 4.8, and 4.9).

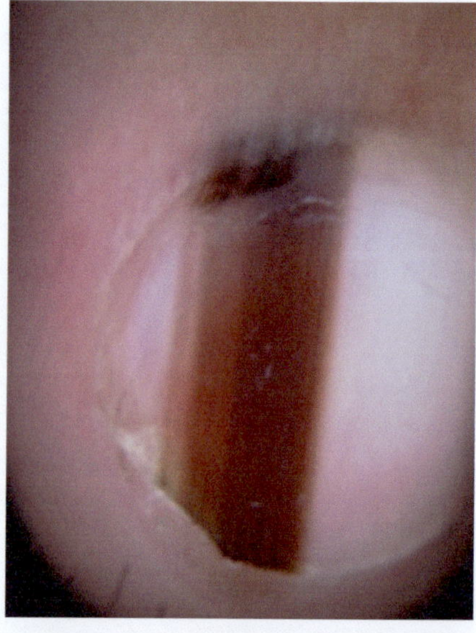

Fig. 4.7 Nevus: band is asymmetric in color distribution, but individual lines are regular in spacing and parallelism, and maintain regular color throughout its longitudinal growth

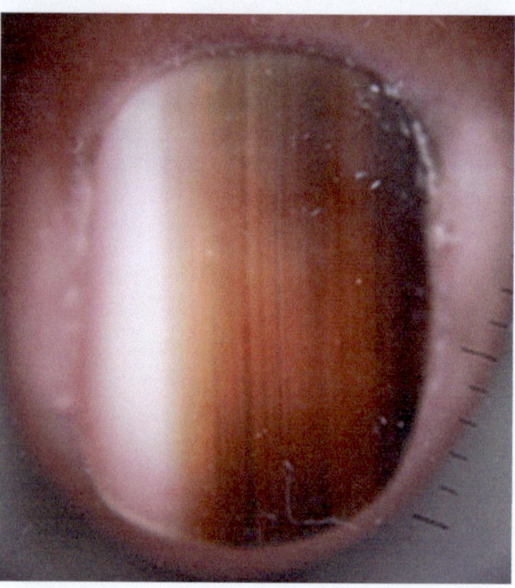

Fig. 4.8 Nevus: *brown* band with regular lines. Again, regularity must be considered regarding each individual line

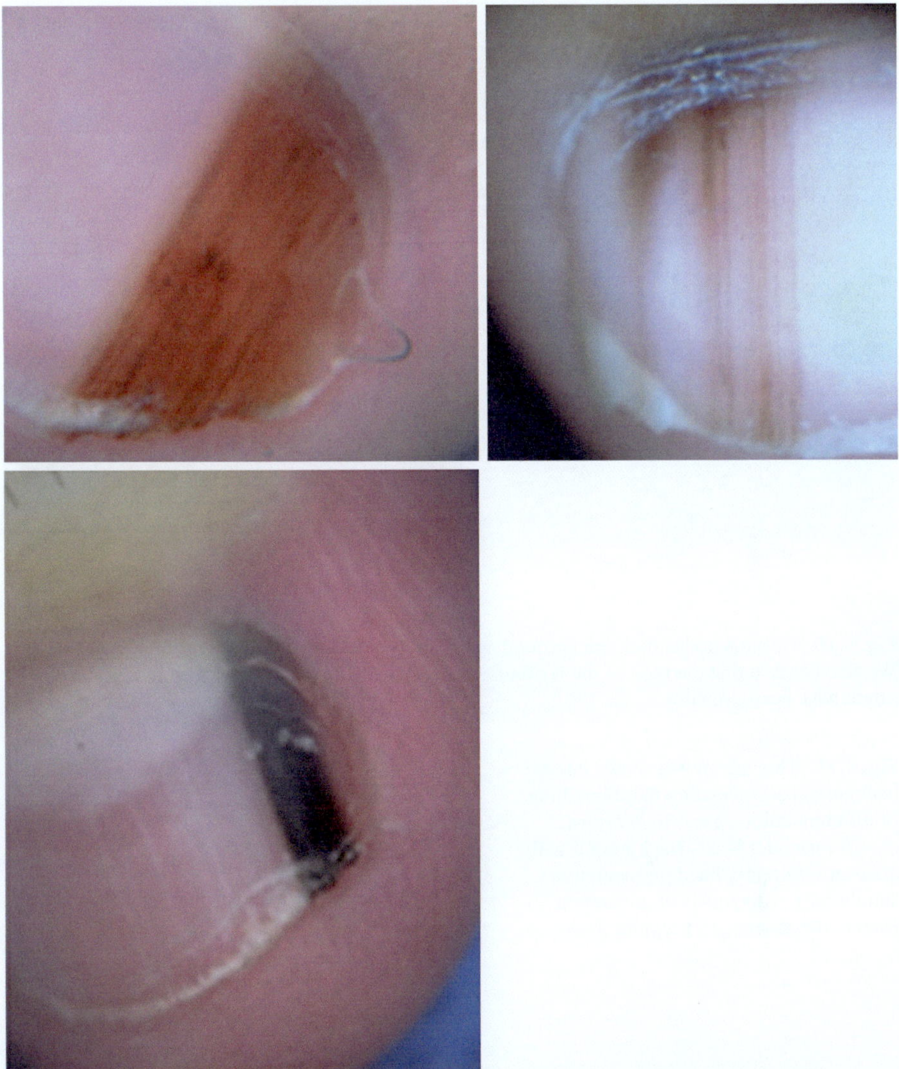

Fig. 4.9 Benign nevi in children: irregular clinical and dermoscopic patterns are frequently seen

Melanoma of the Nail Matrix

Melanomas are characterized by the presence of brown or black background coloration of the strip on dermoscopy. The lines are irregular (irregular pattern), with different hues of pigmentation – from light brown to black – varying in thicknesses and spacing. The parallelism is disrupted, and sometimes ends suddenly (Ronger et al. 2002) (Figs. 4.10 and 4.11).

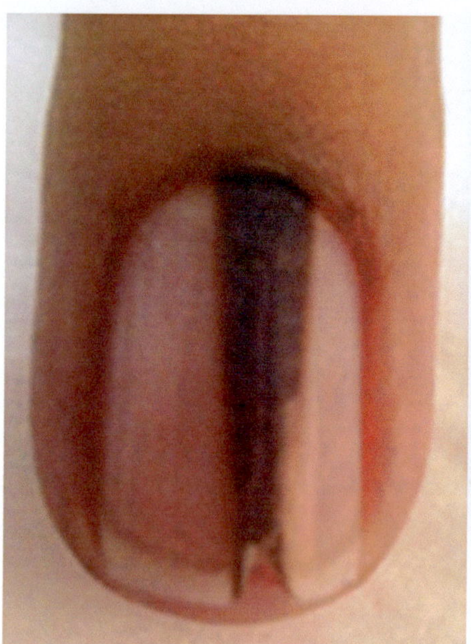

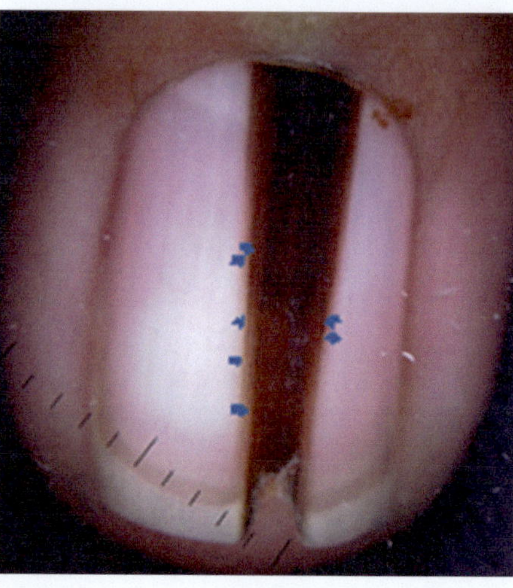

Fig. 4.10 Homogeneous dark background with barely visible lines and globules (*blue arrows*). We also observe that the base of the lesion is wider than the distal part, suggesting that this lesion might have been growing

Fig. 4.11 This melanoma shows intense background pigmentation that blurs lines of different colors: *gray*, *light brown*, *dark brown*, and *black*. Background with areas of differently hued pigmentation should raise a diagnosis of melanoma, even in the absence of irregular lines

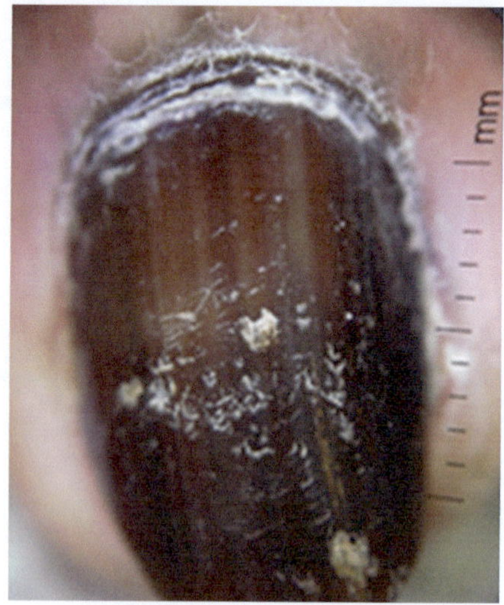

Differential Diagnosis

Subungual Hematoma

Nail plate dermoscopy is very useful for distinguishing blood from melanin. Globular patterns, distal streaks, with a range of color varying from red to brown to black, peripheral fading and periungual hemorrhages are observed (Haenssle et al. 2014) (Fig. 4.12).

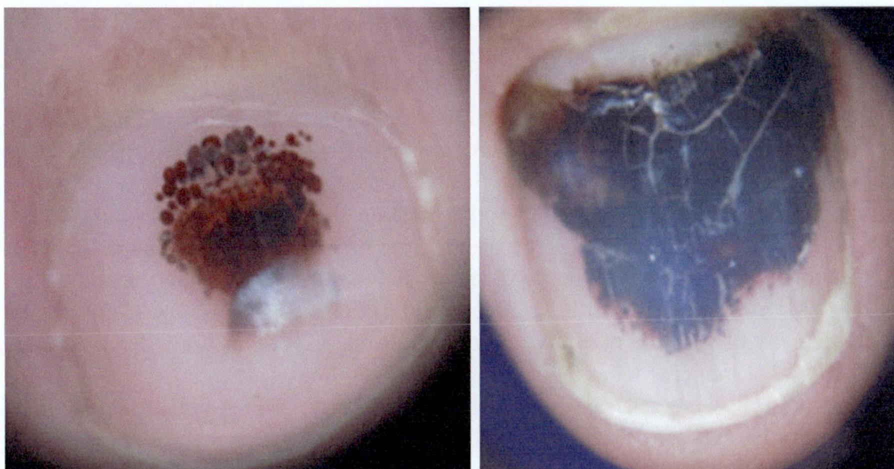

Fig. 4.12 On the *right*, globular red structures and a homogeneous dark red pattern near a leuk-onychia – probably marking trauma location. On the *left*, we observe a central dark homogeneous pattern; *red* dots and globules and distal streaks are seen at the periphery. Clues regarding subungual hemorrhage are often seen at the lesion borders

Fig. 4.13 Onychomycosis: multicolored pattern where we can see a *brown* background pigmentation with *brown–black*, *white*, and *yellow–orange* irregular blotches and streaks

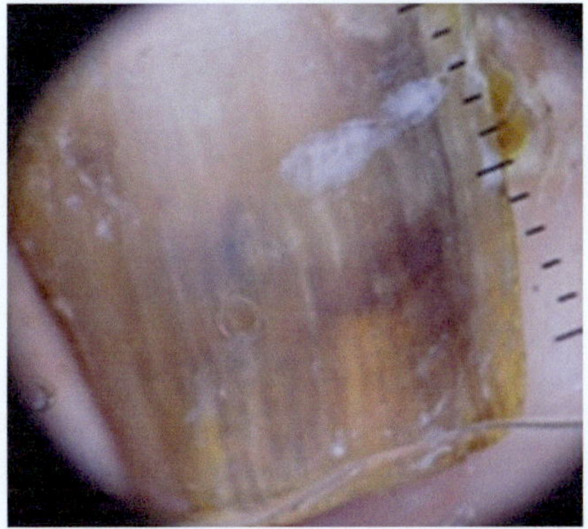

Onychomycosis

In cases of onychomycosis, dermoscopy examination shows a multicolored pattern (black, white, or yellow to brown pigmentation), black pigment aggregates, black reverse triangle, superficial transverse striation, and blurred appearance of pigmentation. Jagged proximal edges with spikes are also frequently observed (Haenssle et al. 2014) (Fig. 4.13).

Pigmented Bowen's Disease

Typical brownish dots along imaginary lines can frequently be observed (Haenssle et al. 2014).

Dermoscopy of the Nail Matrix and Nail Bed

Dermoscopy of the nail matrix and bed (DNMB) is an additional tool for the management of LM. It is indicated when clinical data and dermoscopy of the nail plate do not rule out the possibility of a malignant lesion and a surgical approach is needed (Di Chiacchio et al. 2013b).

Dermoscopy of the nail matrix and bed is an intraoperative procedure where dermoscopy is performed after retraction of the proximal nail fold and removal of the interposed nail plate, allowing direct visualization of pigmented lesions from which LM originates (Hirata et al. 2005, 2006). Polarized light dermoscopy is used to avoid contact with the operative field, permitting a more accurate diagnosis and better surgical management.

Four patterns were described for DNMB (Hirata et al. 2011) of pigmented lesions and are similar to those for nail plate dermoscopy. These patterns correlate well with histological findings and showed high sensitivity and specificity for differentiating melanocytic activation, benign melanocytic hyperplasia, and melanoma. A survey performed by Di Chiacchio et al. (2010) demonstrated that intraoperative dermoscopy was the only factor that statistically improved diagnosis, independent of the examiner's experience, compared with clinical evaluation, the ABCDEF rule for nail melanoma, and dermoscopy of the nail plate.

History

Dermoscopy of the nail bed and matrix was described for the diagnosis of LM by Hirata et al. in 2004 (2006). In this ten-case series the authors demonstrated that analyzing LM at the site of origin revealed characteristics not visualized by nail plate dermoscopy. In a later study (Hirata et al. 2005), they stated that benign and malignant lesions with irregular nail plate dermoscopy had different intraoperative dermoscopic patterns. Finally, in 2011 (Hirata et al. 2011) in a 100-case series of LM (with 15 malignant lesions) Hirata et al. described and validated four dermoscopic patterns with histological correlation. These intraoperative dermoscopic patterns were shown to statistically enhance diagnostic accuracy, for nail experts and general dermatologists, in comparison with clinical evaluation and dermoscopy of the nail plate.

Clinical Features

Intraoperative DNMB

To perform DNMB, a surgical procedure is required to assess the nail matrix and nail bed located underneath the proximal nail fold (Albom 1977; Richert et al. 2011; Scher 1978).

After a distal digital block and placing a tourniquet, we begin detaching the proximal nail fold (PNF) and making a cut longitudinally in both sides of the PNF with a 15 blade. After reclining the proximal nail fold with hooks, we carefully detach the nail plate from the nail bed, using a dental spatula at the back of the nail. The entire nail may be detached but one-third of the proximal nail plate is generally enough for it to be cut transversally and expose the lesion at the nail matrix (Di Chiacchio et al. 2013b). Using a polarized light dermoscope, without contact with the surgical field, we take digital photographs for greater magnification and a more detailed analysis of the pigmented lesion (Fig. 4.14).

Patterns of DNMB Observed According the Diagnosis of LM

Hypermelanosis
A regular gray pattern is seen on the dermoscopy of hypermelanosis (Hirata et al. 2011). It may appear as a homogeneous gray pattern (Hirata et al. 2006) or with discrete gray lines without globules (Hirata et al. 2011). Melanocytic activation on the basal layer, with no evidence for melanocytic proliferation or nests, results in gray or light brown color of the lesion (Hirata et al. 2011) (Fig. 4.15).

Lentigo
A regular brown pattern is indicative of benign hyperplasia. In lentigines we can observe regular lines (according to color, parallelism, spacing, and thickness) without globules or blotches (Hirata et al. 2011). An increased number of typical melanocytes at the basal layer leads to increased production of melanin and is responsible for this regular brown pattern (Hirata et al. 2011) (Figs. 4.16 and 4.17).

Nail Matrix Nevus
In melanocytic nevi, the regular brown pattern appears as regular lines with globules and blotches of regular size and distribution (Hirata et al. 2011). Histologically, these globules and blotches are nests of typical melanocytes and compact aggregates of melanin respectively (Hirata et al. 2011) (Figs. 4.18, 4.19 and 4.20).

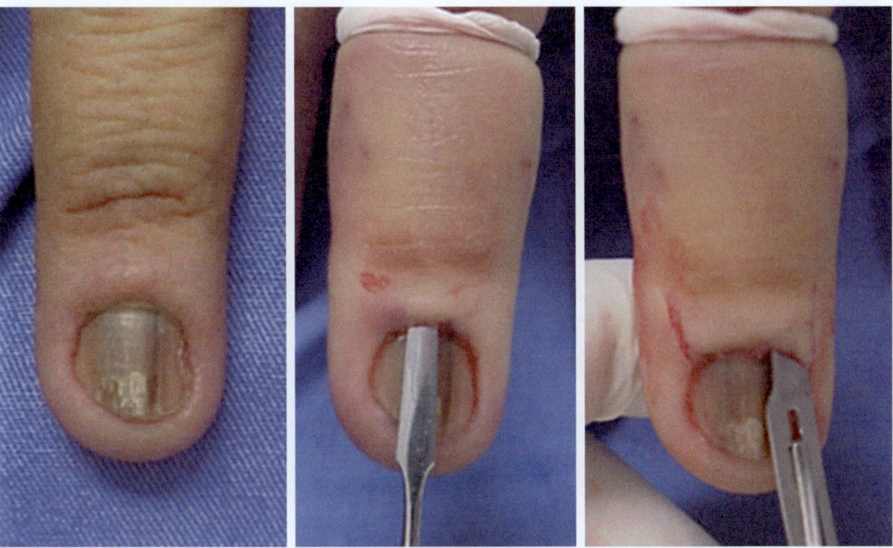

Fig. 4.14 Surgical procedure to assess the nail matrix and nail bed

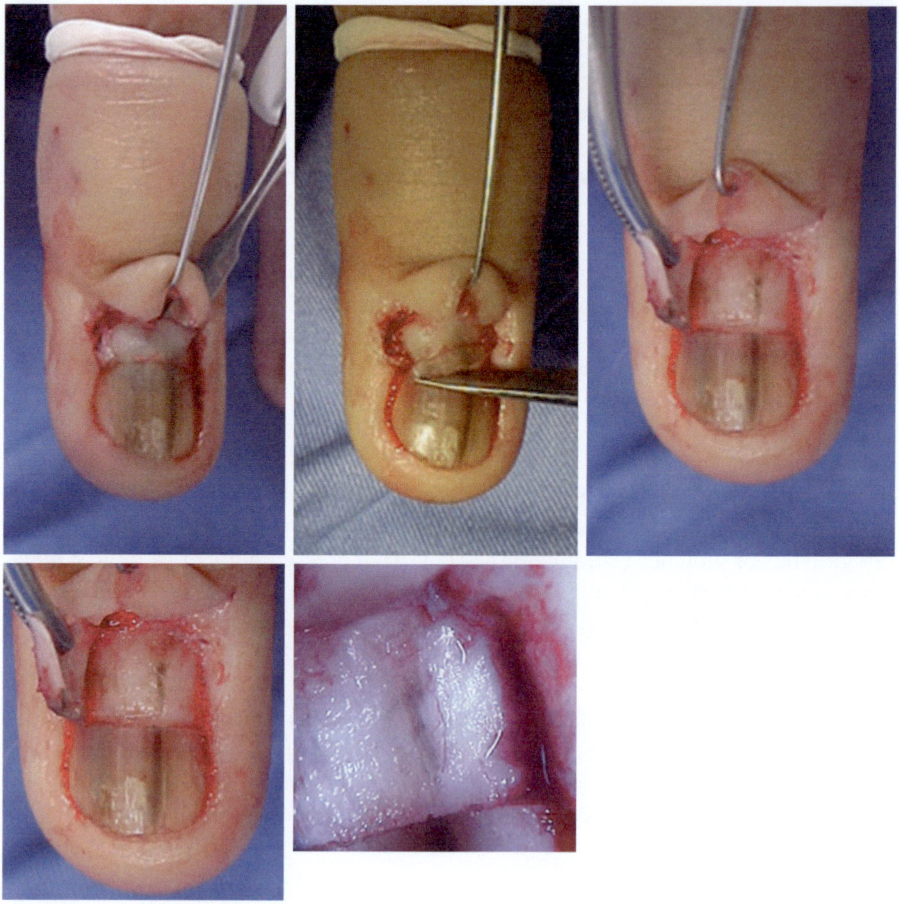

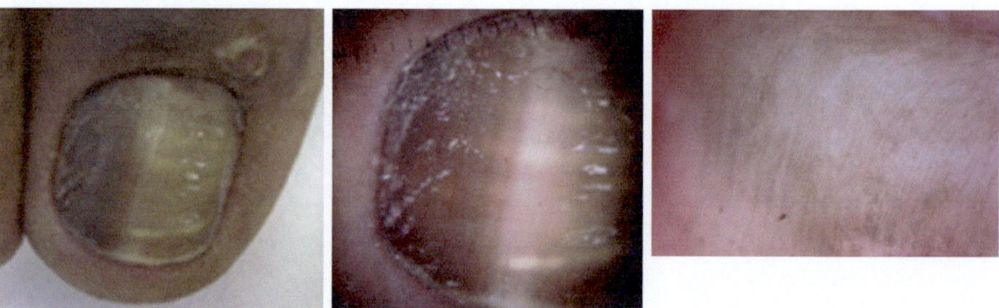

Fig. 4.14 (continued)

Fig. 4.15 Intraoperative dermoscopy showing a regular pattern with *thin gray lines*

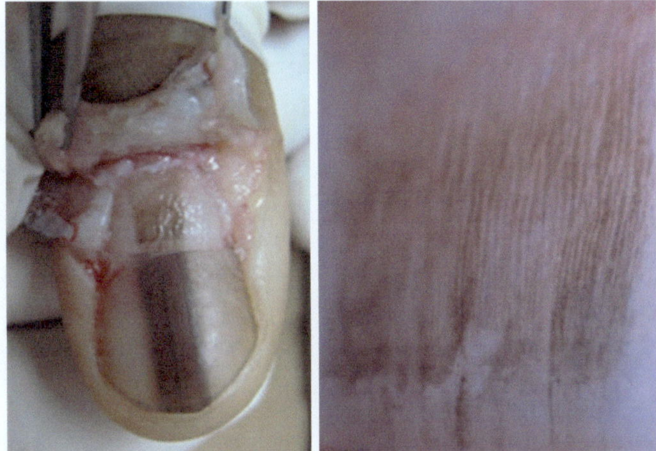

Fig. 4.16 Intraoperative dermoscopy of lentigo showing a regular *brown* pattern with *dark brown/black* parallel lines

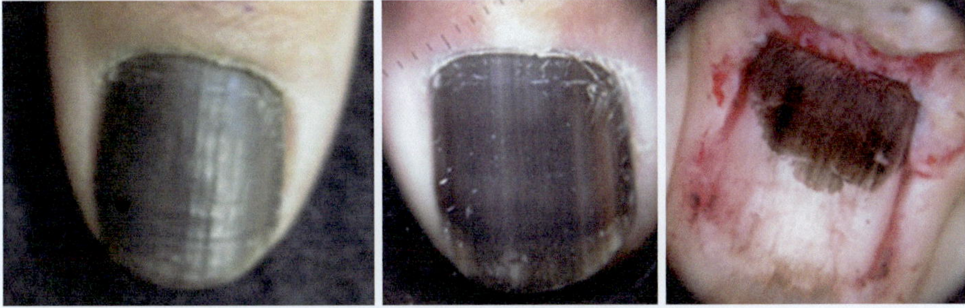

Fig. 4.17 Intraoperative dermoscopy of a lentigo showing a regular *brown* pattern with *dark brown/black* parallel lines

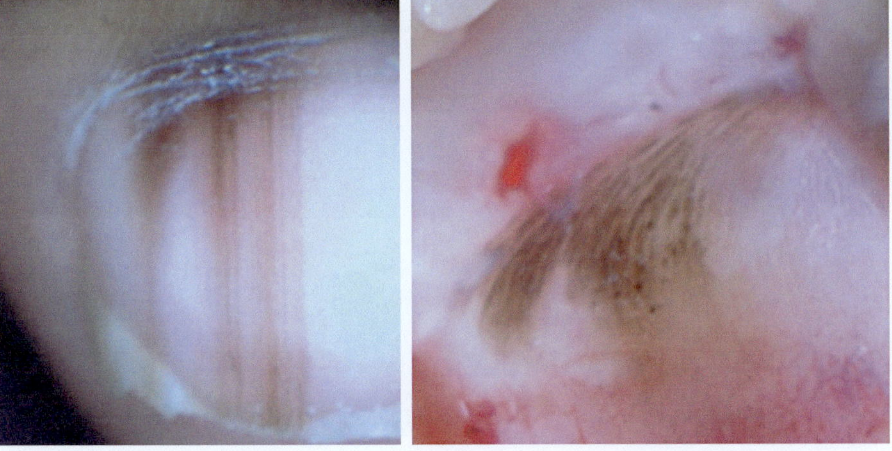

Fig. 4.18 Child with LM and irregular *brown* lines on dermoscopy of the nail plate. Intraoperative dermoscopy showing a regular *brown* pattern with parallel lines and globules

Fig. 4.19 Intraoperative dermoscopy of a nevus showing a regular *brown* pattern with *brown* lines and globules a

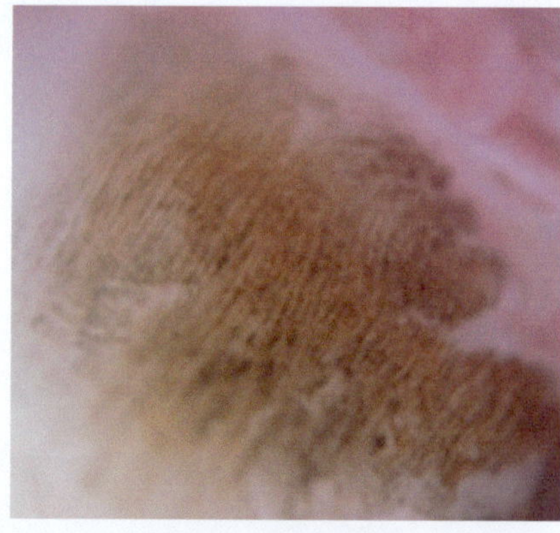

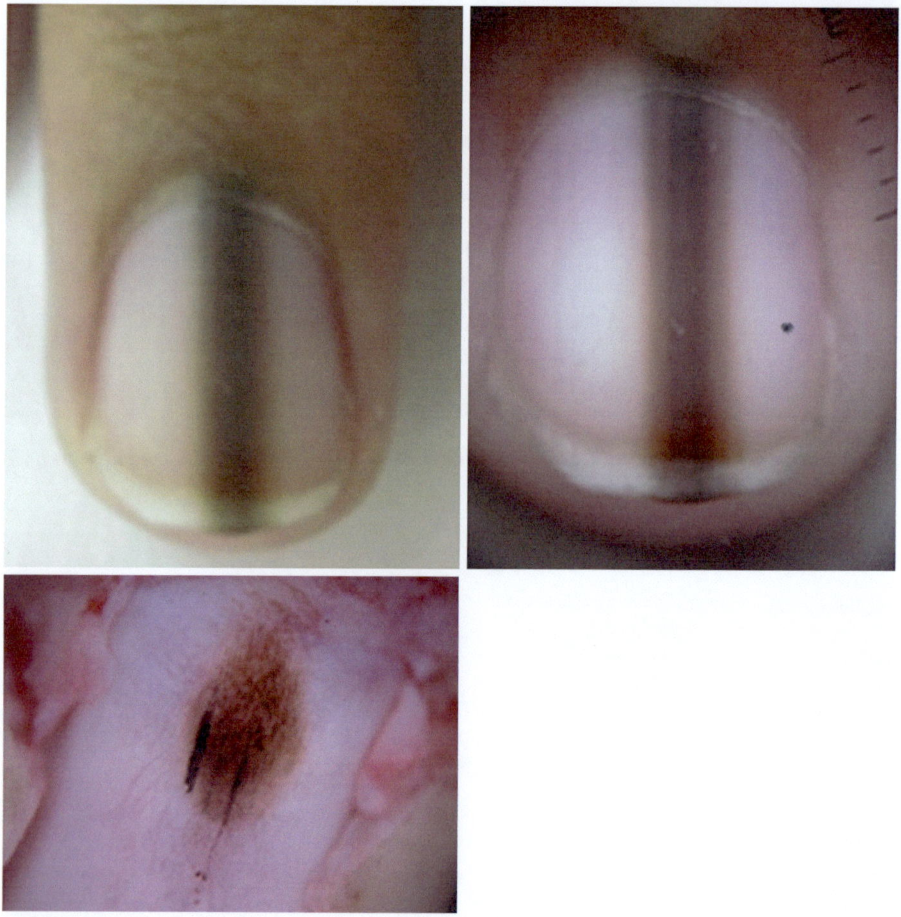

Fig. 4.20 Intraoperative dermoscopy of a nevus showing a global pattern with *brown* lines and globules

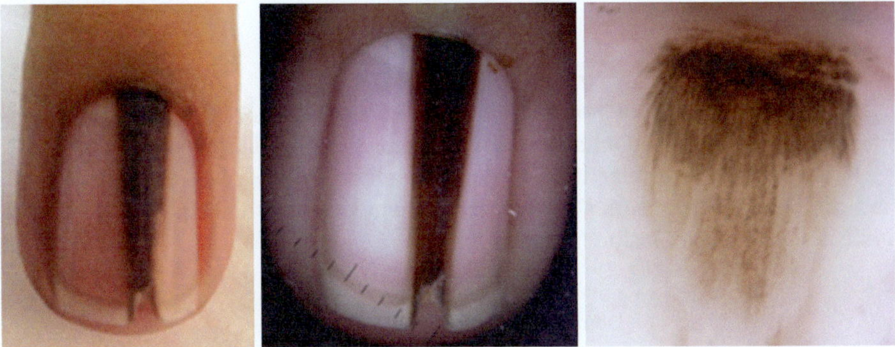

Fig. 4.21 Intraoperative dermoscopy of a melanoma showing an irregular *brown* pattern with a *dark brown* blotch and *brown* lines; distally, we can see a *dotted* pattern with a few globules

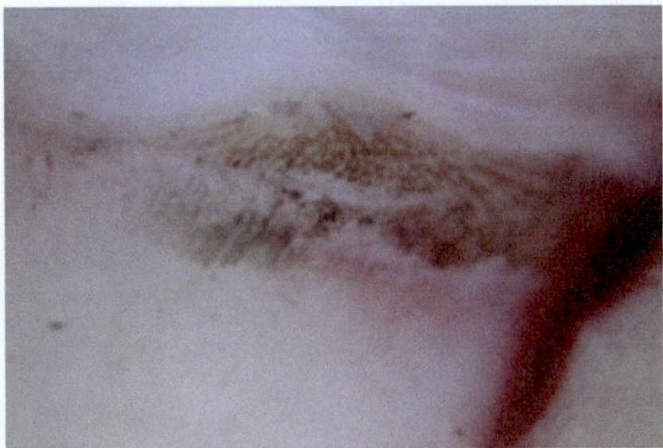

Fig. 4.22 Intraoperative dermoscopy of a melanoma showing an irregular *brown* pattern with a honeycomb-like network associated with *gray/black* lines, dots, and globules, and *brown* lines; distally, we can see a *dotted* pattern with a few globules

Blue Nevi of the Nail Matrix

To our knowledge, only one case of blue nevus has been published with a description of DNMB (Göktay et al. 2015). A rather irregular pattern is observed with a central heavily pigmented blotch and irregular globules, extending linearly to the nail bed with gray–black dots and globules.

Melanoma of the Nail Matrix

Presence of an irregular pattern of colors, lines, globules, and blotches (Hirata et al. 2011). A chaotic pattern containing streaks, globules, dots, structureless areas, and brown–black pigmentation (Hirata et al. 2005) was also described as a multicomponent pattern, similar to that reported for skin melanomas (Figs. 4.21 and 4.22).

Diagnostic Clues

A two-step algorithm may be used to evaluate DNMB.

First, we identify the color of the lesion: gray indicates melanocytic activation (hypermelanosis) whereas a predominantly brown color indicates melanocytic hyperplasia.

Next, we must determine if the brown lesion has regular structures in shape, size, and distribution that favor a benign lesion, whereas an irregular, chaotic pattern indicates a malignant lesion (Schema 4.2).

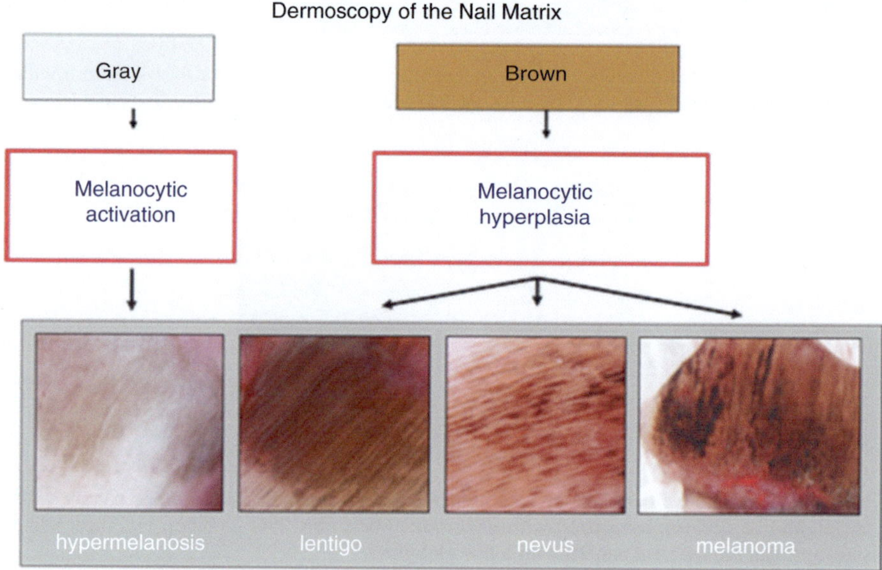

Schema 4.2 Patterns of intraoperative dermoscopy. Gray color means melnocytic activation suggesting hypermelanosis. Brown color means melanocytic hyperplasia. Brown regular lines suggest lentigo, brown regular lines with dots and blotches suggest nevus, and brown irregular lines suggest melanoma

Summary for the Clinician

Intraoperative dermoscopy of the nail matrix is a useful tool for the management of difficult cases of LM. Although some training is needed to perform the surgical technique, the same steps are needed for biopsy and excision of pigmented lesions originating LM. The four main patterns described for dermoscopy of the nail matrix and bed have been shown to have good histological correlation and excellent interobserver reliability between dermatologists. In our experience, intraoperative dermoscopy helps to determine surgical margins for excision and the best location for an incisional biopsy when indicated, but it does not replace histological examination, which remains the gold standard for diagnosis (Jellinek 2010).

References

Albom MJ. Surgical gems: avulsion of a nail plate. J Dermatol Surg Oncol.1977;3(1):34–35.

Baran R, Kechijian P. Longitudinal melanonychia (melanonychia striata): diagnosis and management. J Am Acad Dermatol. 1989;21(6):1165–1175.

Braun RP, Baran R, Le Gal FA, Dalle S, Ronger S, Pandolfi R, et al. Diagnosis and management of nail pigmentations. J Am Acad Dermatol.2007;56(5):835–847.

Di Chiacchio N, Hirata S, Enokihara M, Michalany NS, Fabbrocini G, Tosti A. Dermatologists' accuracy in early diagnosis of melanoma of the nail matrix. Arch Dermatol. 2010;146(4):382–7.

Di Chiacchio N, Ruben BS, Loureiro WR. Longitudinal melanonychias. Clin Dermatol.2013a;31(5): 594–601.

Di Chiacchio ND, de Farias, DC, Piraccini BM, Hirata SH, Richert B, Zaiac M, et al. Consensus on melanonychia nail plate dermoscopy. An Bras Dermatol. 2013b;88(2):309–313.

Göktay F, Güneş P, Yaşar Ş, Güder H, Aytekin S. New observations of intraoperative dermoscopic features of the nail matrix and bed in longitudinal melanonychia. Int J Dermatol. 2015;54(10):1157–62.

Haenssle HA, Blum A, Hofmann-Wellenhof R, Kreusch J, Stolz W, Argenziano G, et al. When all you have is a dermatoscope – start looking at the nails. Dermatol Pract Concept. 4(4):11–20.

Hirata SH, Yamada S, Almeida FA, Tomomori-Yamashita J, Enokihara MY, Paschoal FM, et al. Dermoscopy of the nail bed and matrix to assess melanonychia striata. J Am Acad Dermatol. 2005;53(5):884–6.

Hirata SH, Yamada S, Almeida FA, Enokihara MY, Rosa IP, Enokihara MMS, et al. Dermoscopic examination of the nail bed and matrix. Int J Dermatol. 2006;45(1):28–30.

Hirata SH, Yamada S, Enokihara MY, Di Chiacchio N, de Almeida FA, Enokihara MMSS, et al. Patterns of nail matrix and bed of longitudinal melanonychia by intraoperative dermatoscopy. J Am Acad Dermatol. 2011;65(2):297–303.

Jellinek NJ. Dermoscopy between the lines. Arch Dermatol. 2010;146(4):431–3.

Johr RH, Izakovic J. Dermatoscopy/ELM for the evaluation of nail-apparatus pigmentation. Dermatol Surg. 2001;27(3):315–22.

Kawabata Y, Ohara K, Hino H, Tamaki K. Two kinds of Hutchinson's sign, benign and malignant. J Am Acad Dermatol. 2001;44(2):305–7.

Lazaridou E, Giannopoulou C, Fotiadou C, Demiri E, Ioannides D. Congenital nevus of the nail apparatus – diagnostic approach of a case through dermoscopy. Pediatr Dermatol. 2013;30(6):e293–4.

Marghoob AA, Malvehy J, Braun RP, Kopf AW. An atlas of dermoscopy. Boca Raton : CRC Press; 2004.

Piraccini BM, Dika E, Fanti PA. Tips for diagnosis and treatment of nail pigmentation with practical algorithm. Dermatol Clin. 2015;33(2):185–95.

Richert B, Di Chiacchio N, Haneke E. Nail surgery. 1st ed. New York: CRC Press; 2011 .204 p

Ronger S, Touzet S, Ligeron C, Balme B, Viallard AM, Barrut D, et al. Dermoscopic examination of nail pigmentation. Arch Dermatol. 2002;138(10):1327–33.

Scher RK. Punch biopsies of nails: a simple, valuable procedure. J Dermatol Surg Oncol. 1978;4(7):528–30.

Hypermelanosis (Melanocyte Activation)

5

Brian E. Bishop and Antonella Tosti

Key Features
- Melanonychia due to melanocyte activation may present as a longitudinal, horizontal, or diffuse band of gray, brown, or black pigmentation extending from the nail matrix to the free margin of the nail plate.
- Hypermelanosis is responsible for the majority of adult cases of longitudinal melanonychia, especially in patients with darker skin phototypes.
- Hypermelanosis is defined by increased melanin production and pigmentation of the nail matrix epithelium and nail plate without an increase in the number of melanocytes on histological examination.
- Most etiologies of hypermelanosis are benign and can be identified by a thorough history and physical examination.
- Failure to identify a cause of melanonychia should raise concern with regard to nail apparatus melanoma and requires histopathological evaluation.

Introduction

Melanonychia typically appears as a longitudinal band (longitudinal melanonychia, LM) of gray, brown, or black nail plate pigmentation extending from the nail matrix to the free margin of the nail plate. It is a clinical finding that is often diagnostically challenging owing to the myriad of benign and malignant etiologies associated with its presentation. Melanocytic activation (hypermelanosis) is

B.E. Bishop, BS (✉) • A. Tosti, MD
Department of Dermatology and Cutaneous Surgery, University of Miami Leonard M. Miller School of Medicine, Miami, FL, USA
e-mail: antonellatosti@hotmail.com

© Springer International Publishing Switzerland 2017
N. Di Chiacchio, A. Tosti (eds.), *Melanonychias*,
DOI 10.1007/978-3-319-44993-7_5

responsible for the majority of LM cases in adults and is typically associated with benign etiologies (Haneke and Baran 2001; Andre and Lateur 2006). Hypermelanosis occurs as a result of increased melanin production and pigmentation of the nail matrix epithelium and nail plate, without an increase in the number of melanocytes (Jefferson and Rich 2012). A variety of local and systemic factors, including local trauma, drugs, inflammation, pathogens, neoplasms, and system illness, may activate the normally quiescent melanocytes of the nail matrix (Baran and Kechijian 1989). Although the overwhelming majority of hypermelanosis etiologies are benign, nail apparatus melanoma is a frequently misdiagnosed cause of LM that is associated with a significant delay in diagnosis and a very poor prognosis (Tosti et al. 2009; Klausner et al. 1987). Therefore, it is imperative to distinguish benign causes of hypermelanosis from nail apparatus melanoma in all patients who present with melanonychia.

Epidemiology

Melanocytic activation is responsible for approximately 73% of all adult cases of single-digit LM (Tosti et al. 1996). It is much more prevalent in individuals with darker skin phototypes and typically affects older adults (Baran and Kechijian 1989; Duhard et al. 1995). Physiologic or "racial" hypermelanosis affects approximately 77% of African–Americans over the age of 20, nearly 100% of African–Americans over the age of 50, and roughly 10–20% of all Japanese adults (Baran and Kechijian 1989). Furthermore, it accounts for 68.6% of LM cases within the Hispanic population (Dominguez-Cherit et al. 2008). LM is uncommon among Caucasian adults, where it affects approximately 1.4% of the population (Duhard et al. 1995).

The incidence of LM may also be associated with increasing age (Duhard et al. 1995; Leung et al. 2007). In a study of 4,400 patients, the incidence of LM progressively increased with age and was most prevalent among patients 45–65 years of age (Duhard et al. 1995).

History

Higashi first demonstrated the presence of DOPA-positive melanocytes in the normal nail matrix in 1968 (Higashi 1968). Higashi and Saito subsequently confirmed that the distribution and number of DOPA-positive melanocytes in the nail matrix differed from those in the normal epidermis in size and number. Melanocytes in the distal nail matrix were larger and more numerous compared with the proximal matrix with a distal DOPA-positive melanocyte density ranging from 208 to 576 cells/mm^2 (Higashi and Saito 1969). Hashimoto's ultrastructural study further verified the presence of melanocytes in normal nails by identifying multiple dendritic melanocytes in the nail matrices of white, Japanese, and black individuals. In this particular study, recognizable melanosomes were occasionally found in white persons and consistently found in black and Japanese persons (Hashimoto 1971; Tosti et al. 1994).

Clinical Features

Hypermelanosis typically appears as an asymptomatic longitudinal band of gray, brown, or black nail plate pigmentation extending from the nail matrix to the tip of the nail plate (Fig. 5.1). Rarely, it may appear as a transverse band of pigmentation (transverse melanonychia) or pigmentation of the entire nail plate (total melanonychia). Hypermelanosis commonly involves multiple nails and may present with a variety of additional symptoms depending on its etiology. There are numerous factors associated with melanocytic activation and subsequent nail plate pigmentation that can be categorized as physiological, iatrogenic, traumatic, dermatological, pathogen-induced, or systemic (Tosti et al. 2009).

Physiological Causes

Physiological hypermelanosis is a benign cause of nail plate pigmentation that is frequently seen in patients with dark skin phototypes ("racial" melanonychia) and in pregnancy. It classically presents with single or multiple longitudinal bands of pigmentation involving multiple nails (Fig. 5.2). The number and width of the bands may increase with age (Andre and Lateur 2006; Baran and Kechijian 1989). Pigmented bands typically appear on the nails of digits used for grasping (the thumb, index, and middle fingers) and those prone to trauma (i.e., the big toe) (Andre and Lateur 2006).

Iatrogenic Causes

Phototherapy, X-ray exposure, electron-beam therapy, and medications can cause melanocytic activation and subsequent melanonychia. Patients typically present with

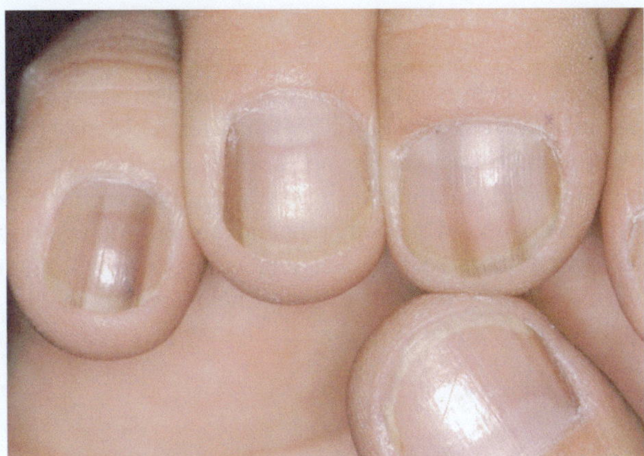

Fig. 5.1 Multiple pale brown bands of linear pigmentation affecting multiple digits

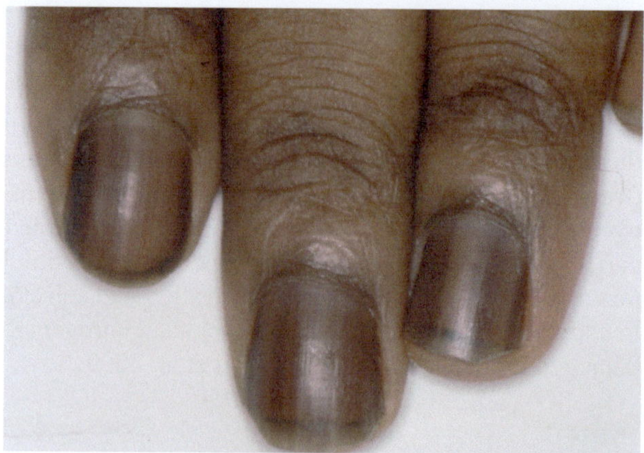

Fig. 5.2 Physiological ("racial") melanonychia involving multiple digits

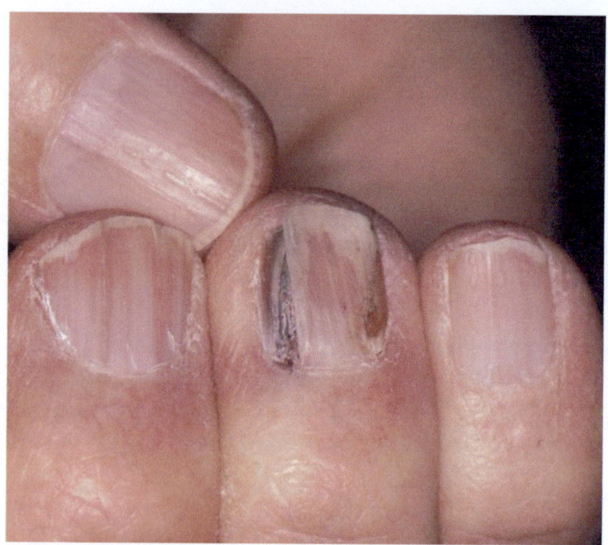

Fig. 5.3 Longitudinal melanonychia secondary to occupational radiation exposure; the patient is a veterinarian. Also note fissuring and onycholysis

multiple light brown-to-black longitudinal or transverse bands affecting multiple fingernails and toenails (Fig. 5.3). However, there may be significant variation in clinical findings depending upon the exposure (Andre and Lateur 2006). Transverse melanonychia, despite being exceedingly rare, is almost exclusive to iatrogenic hypermelanosis. Chemotherapeutic agents are responsible for most documented cases of transverse melanonychia, especially when administered as a multi-drug regimen (Fig. 5.4). Most cases of melanonychia due to iatrogenic causes fade over time with treatment cessation, but it may take years to completely resolve (Piraccini and Tosti 1999).

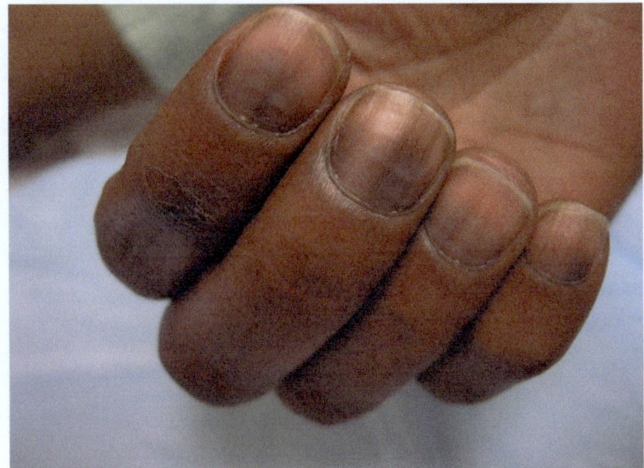

Fig. 5.4 Melanonychia and Muehrcke's lines affecting multiple digits in a patient undergoing chemotherapy

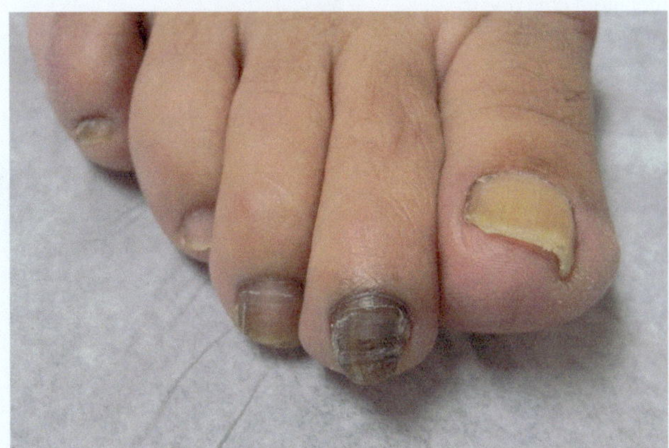

Fig. 5.5 Melanonychia due to trauma; note the associated overriding toe deformity

Local or Regional Causes

Local trauma to the nail plate secondary to onychophagia (nail biting), nail picking, or onychotillomania can also cause melanocytic activation and nail plate pigmentation. Patients commonly present with diffuse bands of melanin pigmentation and signs of associated trauma to the nail plate or periungual tissues (Figs. 5.5 and 5.6). Notable findings include Beau's lines, onychorrhexis, nail thinning, longitudinal striations, cuticular damage and crusts, and splitting of the distal margin, among others (Andre and Lateur 2006; Tosti et al. 2009).

Frictional trauma to the proximal nail fold from poorly fitting shoes or overriding toes may also result in melanocytic activation. It typically presents as brown pigmentation of the nail over the medial aspect of the great toe and lateral aspects of

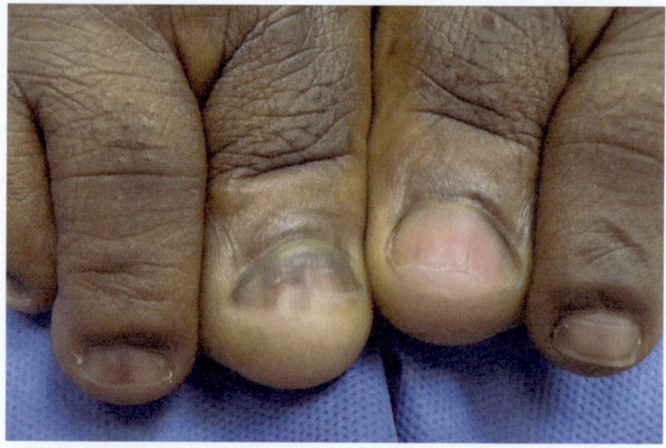

Fig. 5.6 Melanonychia secondary to onychotillomania: note nail thinning and splinters

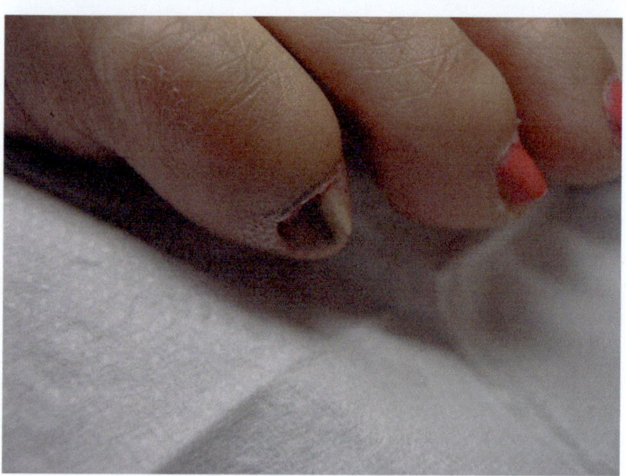

Fig. 5.7 Longitudinal melanonychia due to frictional insult

the fourth and fifth toes (Fig. 5.7). It usually appears in a symmetrical distribution and may affect part of the nail or the entire nail. The affected digit may present with anatomical abnormalities indicative of trauma (Tosti et al. 2009).

Dermatological Causes

Dermatological conditions such as psoriasis, Hallopeau's acrodermatitis, lichen planus, amyloidosis, paronychia, and chronic radiodermatitis can also cause hypermelanosis. Inflammatory changes in the nail plate induce melanocytic activation and subsequent melanin production. These patients typically present with a single light-brown longitudinal band of pigmentation that appears shortly after the resolution of an inflammatory process (Fig. 5.8). The pigmented bands may lighten and eventually resolve over time with treatment of the underlying inflammatory process (Andre and Lateur 2006).

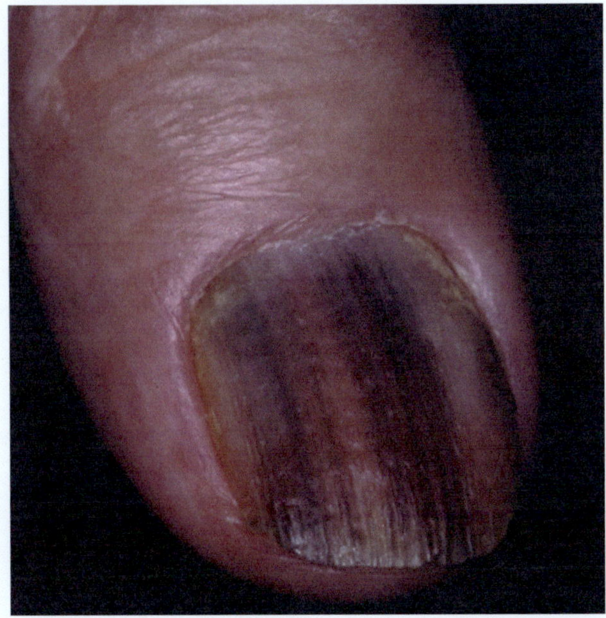

Fig. 5.8 Post-inflammatory bands of melanonychia in a patient with Hallopeau's acrodermatitis

Pathogenic Causes

Various pathogenic organisms may also cause or mimic melanonychia in affected nails. Onychomycosis can cause melanonychia by triggering an inflammatory response within the nail plate or by directly producing melanin. Patients may present with a single, light-brown longitudinal band of pigmentation, multiple longitudinal bands of pigmentation or a diffuse pattern of pigmentation (Tosti et al. 2009). Diffuse bands of nail pigmentation have also been reported as a result of bacterial (*Proteus mirabilis*) pathogens, nondermatophytic molds (*Neoscytalidium dimidiatum, Alternaria alternate*), and dermatophytic molds (*Trichophyton rubrum* var. *nigricans*) (Perrin and Baran 1994; Romano et al. 1985). Other organisms may also mimic melanonychia by producing nonmelanic dark black or brown pigment.

Systemic Causes

Melanonychia is rare manifestation of systemic pathological conditions that may be associated with endocrine disorders, nutritional disorders, HIV infection, hemosiderosis, alkaptonuria, hyperbilirubinemia, and porphyria. Patients typically develop multiple bands of dark brown pigmentation involving multiple fingernails and toenails. Interestingly, systemic causes of melanonychia also commonly present with associated mucosal or cutaneous pigmentation (Andre and Lateur 2006).

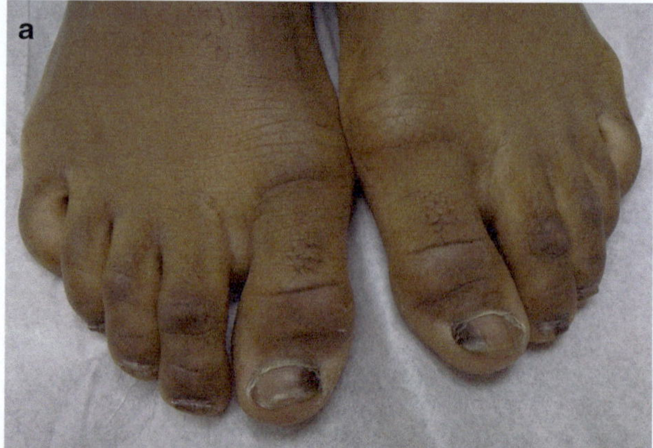

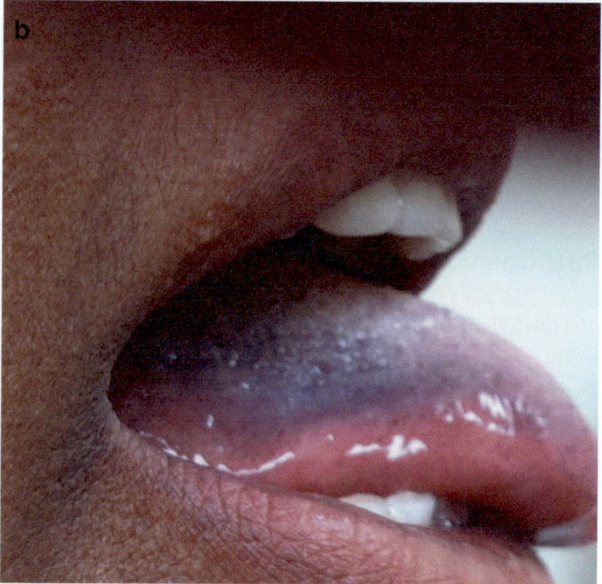

Fig. 5.9 (**a**) Melanonychia of multiple toenails in a patient with Laugier–Hunziker disease, (**b**) Pigmented mucosal macule in a patient with Laugier–Hunziker disease

Syndrome-associated melanonychia occurs in patients with Laugier–Hunziker, Peutz–Jeghers, or Touraine syndromes. Laugier–Hunziker syndrome predominantly affects white individuals between 20 and 40 years of age. Patients typically present with single or multiple bands of longitudinal pigmentation on multiple fingernails and pigmented macules involving the lips and oral cavity (Fig. 5.9). Peutz–Jeghers and Touraine syndromes present with very similar cutaneous and nail manifestations; however, the pigmented macules in these syndromes usually appear during early childhood (Andre and Lateur 2006).

Other Causes

Nonmelanocytic tumors of the nail apparatus, such as onychomatricoma, myxoid pseudocyst, basal cell carcinoma, squamous cell carcinoma, fibrous histiocytoma, and verruca vulgaris, have also been associated with LM secondary to melanocyte activation. These etiologies are exceedingly rare and may present with a longitudinal band of pigmentation aligned with the causative lesion (Andre and Lateur 2006).

Diagnostic Clues

History

The evaluation of patients presenting with nail pigmentation should begin with a thorough history, including the onset, progression, and potential triggers of melanonychia. Information regarding occupation, hobbies, medication/drug exposure, history of local or frictional trauma, medical history, and family history should also be obtained to help identify potential etiologies. It may be helpful to have patients fill out a questionnaire with this information to encourage accurate, thoughtful responses in a timely manner (Jefferson and Rich 2012).

Physical Examination

Physical examination should include evaluation of all 20 nails in addition to the skin and mucous membranes. The fingernails should be examined while resting the patient's hands on a flat surface and the toenails should be examined while the patient is standing and sitting to assess for frictional forces due to overlapping toes or poorly fitting shoes. Evaluation of the nails should include examination of the nail plate and periungual tissues while moving the digit to provide frontal, lateral, and inferior views of the nail.

Dermoscopy

On dermoscopy, melanonychia due to hypermelanosis presents as a gray homogenous band with or without thin regular lines. The presence of dots due to blood extravasation and splinter hemorrhages suggest a traumatic origin (Fig. 5.10).

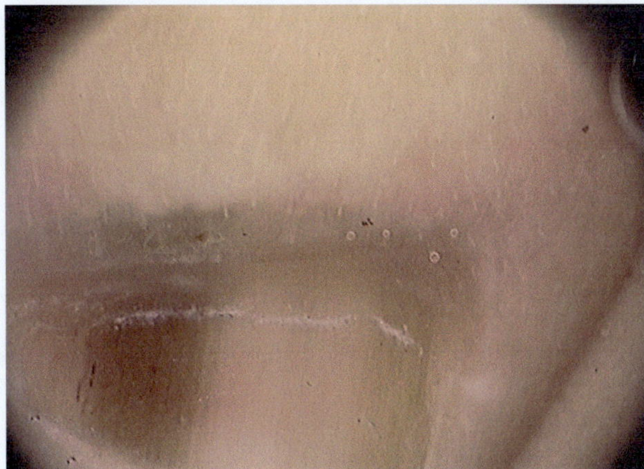

Fig. 5.10 Dermatoscopic findings of melanonychia secondary to frictional trauma, gray uniform band with splinter hemorrhages

Diagnostic Algorithm

The following questions are helpful in guiding the initial examination of nail pigmentation (Fig. 5.11) (Piraccini et al. 2015):

Step 1: Is the pigment due to melanin within the nail?
Melanic nail pigmentation is characterized by gray, brown, or black pigmentation within the nail plate, whereas other forms of nail pigmentation vary in color and localization. It is helpful to use a dermatoscope to evaluate the color of nail pigmentation and rule out other causes of nonmelanic pigmentation, particularly green nails, nonmelanic fungal pigmentation, and subungual hematomas. Gently scraping the pigmented area of the nail can further help to identify whether the pigmentation is localized within the nail plate to rule out exogenous pigmentation.

Step 2: Does melanonychia involve one or several digits?
Hypermelanosis of physiological, iatrogenic, systemic, and frictional causes typically involves multiple nails, whereas local trauma, inflammatory causes, and nail tumors (onychopapilloma, onychomatricoma, Bowen's disease) only affect one digit. Melanonychia due to onychotillomania also tends to affect multiple digits, but may present with single-digit involvement under certain circumstances.

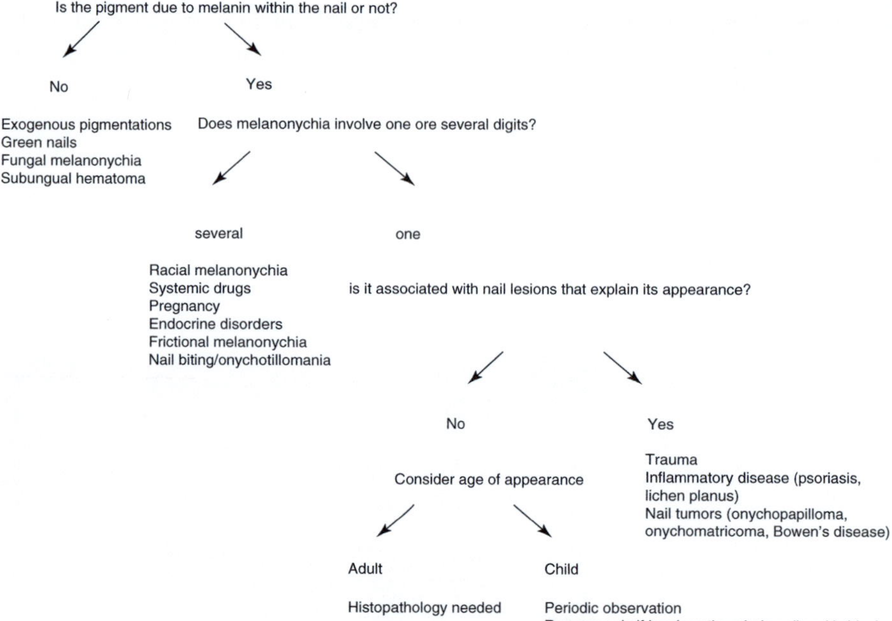

Fig. 5.11 Diagnostic algorithm for the evaluation of nail plate pigmentation (Piraccini et al. 2015)

Step 3: Is it associated with nail lesions that explain its appearance?

Many causes of hypermelanosis are associated with other signs and symptoms that are characteristic of the etiology. It is important to examine the nails for signs of trauma to the nail plate, inflammatory/dermatological disease, or nail tumors. Other associated signs, such as mucosal or cutaneous pigmentation, should also be considered when establishing a diagnosis.

Step 4: Age at appearance?

Age should also be taken into consideration when evaluating nail pigmentation, especially when it only involves one digit. Single-digit LM in children is most commonly caused by a benign nail matrix nevus and can be observed in most cases. In adults, single-digit LM with no identifiable cause is very concerning with regard to nail apparatus melanoma and further histopathology is recommended.

Summary for the Clinician

Longitudinal melanonychia is a relatively common clinical finding with inherent diagnostic challenges owing to the myriad of benign and malignant etiologies. Hypermelanosis is responsible for the majority of cases of LM, especially in patients with darker skin phototypes, and is typically associated with benign etiologies. However, nail apparatus melanoma may also present with LM and is associated with a significant delay in diagnosis and poor prognosis. Therefore, it is imperative to distinguish benign causes of hypermelanosis from nail apparatus melanoma in all patients presenting with LM.

References

Andre J, Lateur N. Pigmented nail disorders. Dermatol Clin. 2006;24(3):329–39.

Baran R, Kechijian P. Longitudinal melanonychia (melanonychia striata): diagnosis and management. J Am Acad Dermatol. 1989;21(6):1165–75.

Dominguez-Cherit J, Roldan-Marin R, Pichardo-Velazquez P, Valente C, Fonte-Avalos V, Vega-Memije ME, Toussaint-Caire S. Melanonychia, melanocytic hyperplasia, and nail melanoma in a Hispanic population. J Am Acad Dermatol. 2008;59(5):785–91.

Duhard E, Calvet C, Mariotte N, Tichet J, Vaillant L. Prevalence of longitudinal melanonychia in the white population. Ann Dermatol Venereol. 1995;122(9):586–90.

Haneke E, Baran R. Longitudinal melanonychia. Dermatol Surg. 2001;27(6):580–4.

Hashimoto K. Ultrastructure of the human toenail. I. Proximal nail matrix. J Invest Dermatol. 1971;56(3):235–46.

Higashi N. Melanocytes of nail matrix and nail pigmentation. Arch Dermatol. 1968;97(5):570–4.

Higashi N, Saito T. Horizontal distribution of the dopa-positive melanocytes in the nail matrix. J Invest Dermatol. 1969;53(2):163–5.

Jefferson J, Rich P. Melanonychia. Dermatol Res Pract. 2012;2012:952186.

Klausner JM, Inbar M, Gutman M, Weiss G, Skornick Y, Chaichik S, Rozin RR. Nail-bed melanoma. J Surg Oncol. 1987;34(3):208–10.

Leung AK, Robson WL, Liu EK, Kao CP, Fong JH, Leong AG, Cheung BC, Wong AH, Chen SY. Melanonychia striata in Chinese children and adults. Int J Dermatol. 2007;46(9):920–2.

Perrin C, Baran R. Longitudinal melanonychia caused by trichophyton rubrum. Histochemical and ultrastructural study of two cases. J Am Acad Dermatol. 1994;31(2 Pt 2):311–6.

Piraccini BM, Tosti A. Drug-induced nail disorders: incidence, management and prognosis. Drug Saf. 1999;21(3):187–201.

Piraccini BM, Dika E, Fanti PA. Tips for diagnosis and treatment of nail pigmentation with practical algorithm. Dermatol Clin. 2015;33(2):185–95.

Romano C, Paccagnini E, Difonzo EM. Onychomycosis caused by Alternaria spp. in Tuscany, Italy from 1985 to 1999. Mycoses. 2001;44(3–4):73–6.

Tosti A, Cameli N, Piraccini BM, Fanti PA, Ortonne JP. Characterization of nail matrix melanocytes with anti-PEP1, anti-PEP8, TMH-1, and HMB-45 antibodies. J Am Acad Dermatol. 1994;31(2 Pt 1):193–6.

Tosti A, Baran R, Piraccini BM, Cameli N, Fanti PA. Nail matrix nevi: a clinical and histopathologic study of twenty-two patients. J Am Acad Dermatol. 1996;34(5 Pt 1):765–71.

Tosti A, Piraccini BM, de Farias DC. Dealing with melanonychia. Semin Cutan Med Surg. 2009;28(1):49–54.

Lentigo and Nevus

6

Eckart Haneke

Key Features
- Melanonychia is the most common and earliest visible sign of a subungual melanoma.
- Melanonychia may be due to melanocyte hyperfunction, lentigines, nevi or malignant melanomas of the nail matrix.
- Whereas functional melanonychia is grayish, melanonychia due to lentigines and nevi usually causes a clear brown to sometimes even black nail color.
- The development of matrix lentigines and nevi in adult Caucasians is uncommon and should raise suspicion.
- Benign lentigines and nevi can be safely diagnosed and in most cases treated by a tangential excision without the risk of post-surgical nail dystrophy.

Introduction

Melanoma is the most serious malignant tumor of the nail unit. A brown streak develops in two-thirds to three-quarters of patients and is often visible for years or even decades before the correct diagnosis is made.

E. Haneke, MD, PhD
Department of Dermatology, Inselspital, University of Bern, Bern, Switzerland

Dermatology Practice Dermaticum, Freiburg, Germany

Centro Dermatol, Inst CUF, Porto, Portugal

Department of Dermatology, Academic Hospital, University of Gent, Ghent, Belgium
e-mail: haneke@gmx.net

© Springer International Publishing Switzerland 2017
N. Di Chiacchio, A. Tosti (eds.), *Melanonychias*,
DOI 10.1007/978-3-319-44993-7_6

History

Lentigines and nevi have long been known to be the main causes of brown streaks in the nail, although most attention was always paid to melanonychia in association with subungual melanomas.

Development

Prevalence

Among the melanocytic causes of melanonychia, lentigines and nevi are the second most frequent melanonychia etiology after functional hypermelanosis. Exact numbers for lentigo- and nevus-derived melanonychia do not exist, but they seem to be rare in the Caucasian population, as demonstrated by the systematic examination of 1,000 consecutive patients revealing eight subungual hematomas, but no melanocytic lesions (Shukla and Hughes 1992). Subungual lentigines and nevi occur both in Caucasians and, probably even more frequently, in Asians (Leung and Woo 2004), and are often a matter of concern for patients and/or their parents. They are rare in Blacks (Libow et al. 1995).

Cause

Melanonychia develops when melanocytes in the matrix produce more melanin than the matrix keratinocytes can physiologically disintegrate. The melanin is transferred into matrix keratinocytes that migrate obliquely upward and distally during nail plate genesis. Thus, lentigines and nevi of the nail bed cannot give rise to a longitudinal melanotic band of the nail, as the nail bed does not produce nail plate, but only a thin horny layer, allowing the nail plate to move over the nail bed while advancing, without losing its firm attachment to the nail bed. In fact, lentigines and nevi of the nail bed seem to be exceedingly rare. Blue nevi do not give rise to a longitudinal brown band either (Vidal et al. 1997; Causeret et al. 2003).

Clinical Pattern

Whereas so-called functional melanonychia is usually light brown and said to have a grayish background, melanonychia due to lentigines and nevi is brownish and the color is more pronounced (Figs. 6.1, 6.2, 6.3, and 6.4). Melanonychia is due to a proliferation of melanocytes of the matrix, either as single cells in lentigines or also displaying nests as in nevi. Usually, longitudinal melanonychia shows regular striations in a symmetrical fashion. Dark brown spots, often arranged linearly, may be seen, particularly under dermatoscopy. The spots represent the migration of nevus cell nests into the nail plate. This phenomenon is not infrequently seen in children, but is also occasionally observed in adults.

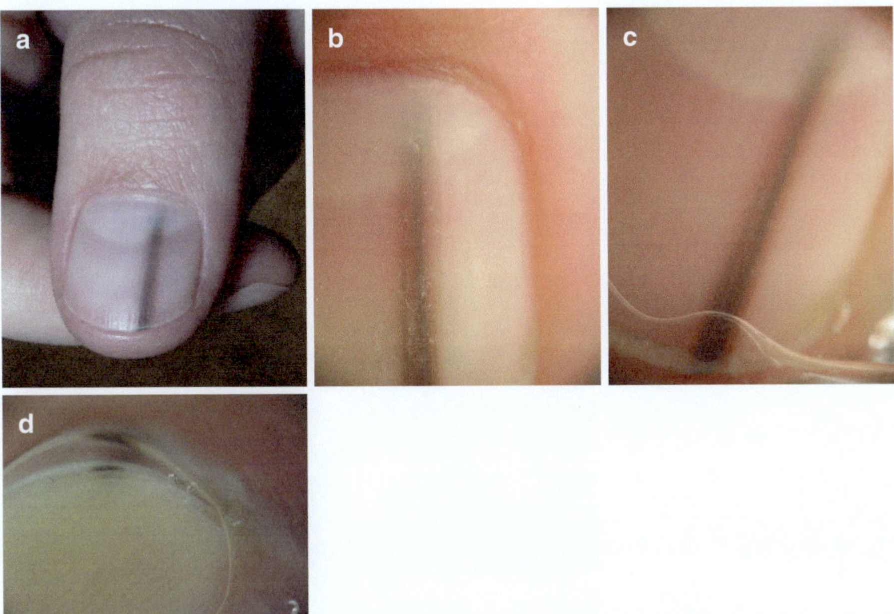

Fig. 6.1 Lentigo of the nail matrix in the thumb nail of a 12-year-old girl causing a regular brown streak in the nail. (**a**) Clinical photo. (**b**) Macrophoto without an optical medium. (**c**) Macrophoto with laser contact gel as an optical medium. (**d**) End-on dermatoscopy shows pigment in the lower half of the nail plate demonstrating its origin from the distal matrix

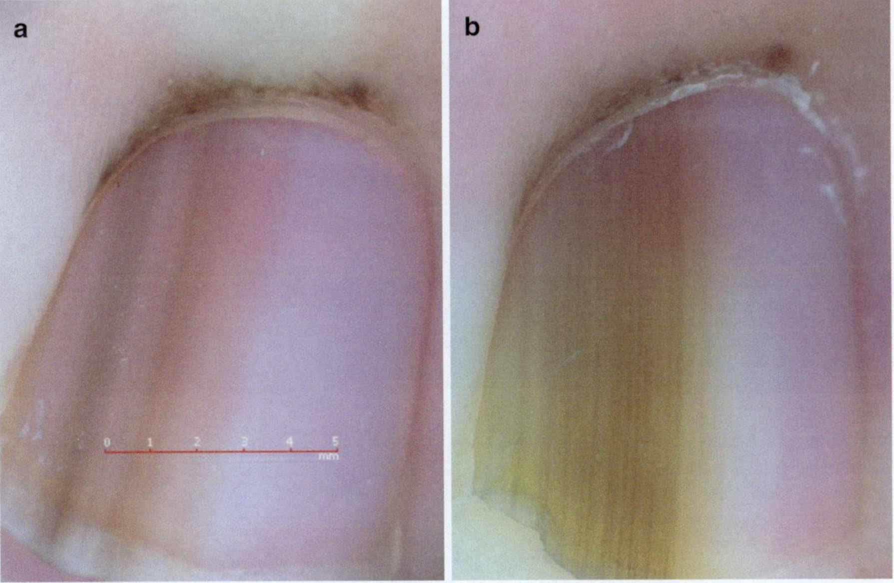

Fig. 6.2 Longitudinal melanonychia in a child showing rapid change in width and periungual pigmentation. (**a**) Clinical presentation at first consultation. (**b**) Presentation 12 weeks later shows a more homogeneous pigmentation with regularly spaced brown lines in the band

Fig. 6.3 Nevus of the matrix of the right little finger nail of a 31-year-old dark-skinned nurse. The brown band is regular, the central portion is darker than the margins

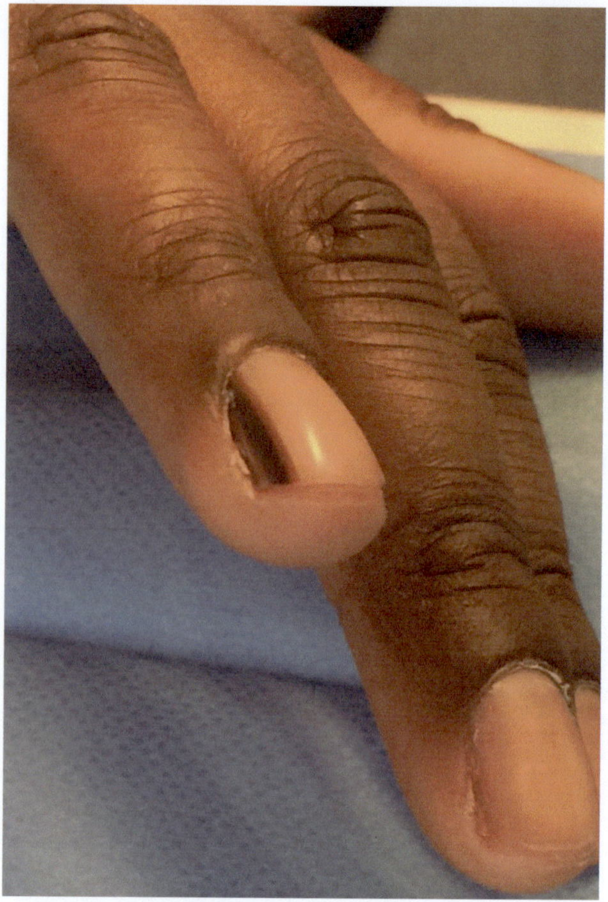

Fig. 6.4 Recurrent matrix nevus in the right ring finger of a 25-year-old woman. A subtotal excision had been performed roughly 2 years before consultation at our department. A homogeneously brown streak is visible in addition to the post-biopsy nail dystrophy. Re-excision by the tangential biopsy method remained without a recurrence after 3 years

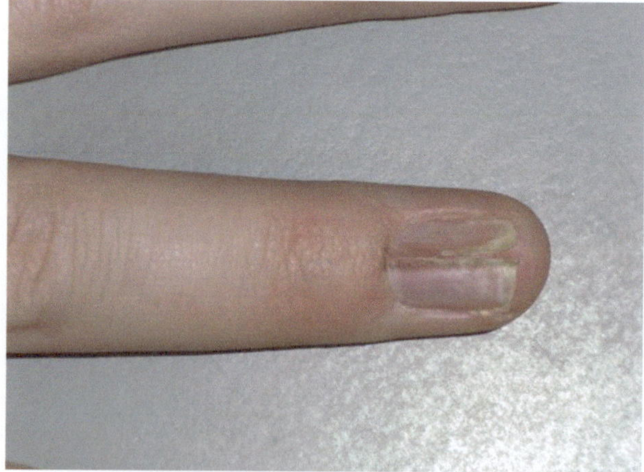

Acquired melanonychia due to lentigines and nevi is usually not wider than 5 mm, although subungual melanomas of 2 mm in diameter have been described (Rosendahl et al. 2012).

Longitudinal melanonychia always runs from the matrix into the free margin of the nail as the melanin is incorporated into the nail substance. It cannot be scraped off like superficial and exogenous pigmentations because of certain bacteria and stains. End-on dermatoscopy usually allows the localization of the melanin within the nail plate to be determined. Pigment in the upper layers is seen when the lentigo or nevus responsible is located in the proximal matrix, in the middle nail layers when it is present in the middle matrix, and in the deep layers when the melanocyte nidus is in the distal matrix; pigment in the entire nail thickness indicates melanocytes from the apical to the distal matrix. Nail clippings stained with Fontana–Masson's argentaffin reaction permit a more precise estimate. Also, other more sophisticated expensive techniques such as optical coherence microscopy and reflectance confocal laser scanning microscopy allow the localization of the melanin to be precisely defined in the nail plate. The latter techniques also enable the investigator to discern nevus cell nests and single melanocytes in the nail plate. Nevus nests can additionally be seen with high-frequency ultrasound.

Significance

Although melanonychia in children is almost invariably benign (Tosti et al. 1996; Léauté-Labrèze et al. 1996; Goettmann-Bonvallot et al. 1999; Theunis et al. 2011), it is always a matter of concern when it arises in adults, particularly in light-skinned individuals, as the underlying cause – simple hypermelanosis, lentigo, nevus or melanoma – cannot be diagnosed with certainty on clinical evidence alone. Dermatoscopy gives a little more accuracy, although criteria such as background color, evenness of striation, regular distance of striae within the band and micro-Hutchinson signs are more easily evaluated.

It has been stated that acquired longitudinal melanonychia in a fair-skinned adult should be seen as malignant rather than benign (Kopf and Waldo 1980). Whereas congenital nevi may give rise to very dark and wide bands, often associated with nevus spread to a part of the surrounding periungual skin, acquired lentigines and nevi of the matrix rarely measure more than 5 mm in diameter. Again, it should be stressed that lentigines and nevi appearing de novo in nonsun-exposed areas beyond the age of 30–40 years are suspicious.

Melanonychia in children often develops rather rapidly, remains stable for years, and then gradually fades to light brown streaks or even disappears completely. In contrast, a brown streak of the nail in a child that after a long stable period rapidly widens is suspicious and requires excisional biopsy with histopathological examination.

In summary, two-thirds to three-quarters of all ungual melanomas start as longitudinal melanonychia (Tomizawa 2000) and thus – theoretically – offer an excellent chance for early diagnosis.

Lentigo and Nevus of the Matrix

Apart from racial pigmentation and melanocyte activation, lentigines and nevi are the most common cause of longitudinal melanonychia. Both are defined as a numerical increase in melanocytes, with single-cell proliferation defining lentigo and at least one nest of melanocytes constituting a nevus. The number of melanocytes is augmented when more than 6.5 melanocytes are seen per millimeter stretch of basal layer (Tosti et al. 1998). In contrast to normal matrix melanocytes that are often localized above the basal row of matrix keratinocytes, melanocytes in lentigines often mainly occupy the basal layer. Immunohistochemically, with special melanin stains, long but slender dendrites can be identified. Nevi display the same characteristics plus nests of melanocytes. These are usually oval and may sometimes be taken up with the maturing cells of the keratogenous zone to finally be included in the nail plate. The degree of pigmentation varies from light brown to almost black; the color intensity does not reflect the dignity of the lesion.

An increase in the number of melanocytes is found in the Laugier–Hunziker–Baran syndrome (Fig. 6.5) (Haneke 1991; Moore et al. 2004), although other authors report a normal number of melanocytes (Makhoul et al. 2003). It may be assumed that the former is also the case in the rare nail involvement in Peutz–Jeghers syndrome (Valero and Sherf 1965).

Congenital nevi sometimes affect the nail unit. They are often much larger than acquired nevi and may involve the entire nail plus periungual tissue, occasionally leading to nail deformation (Ohtsuka et al. 1978; Coskey et al. 1983; Pomerance et al. 1994).

Hutchinson's sign is commonly seen as a reliable marker of ungual melanoma. However, particularly in Japanese subjects, periungual pigmentation has also been observed in benign longitudinal melanonychia (Asahina et al. 1989; Kawabata et al. 2001) and it is not uncommon in congenital melanocytic nevi of the nail (Agusti-Mejias et al. 2013).

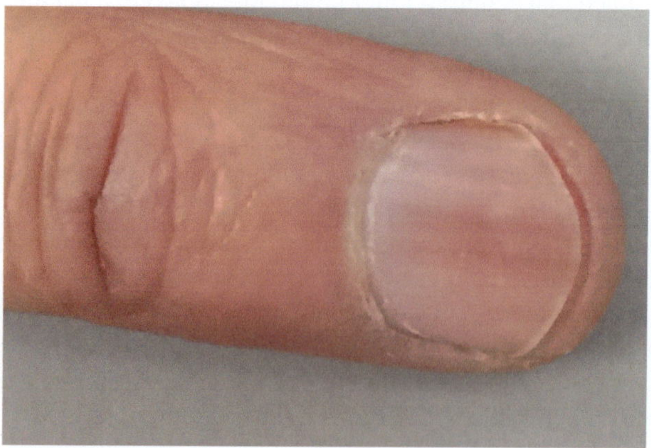

Fig. 6.5 Laugier–Hunziker–Baran syndrome in a 53-year-old female patient

Diagnosis

For the clinical differential diagnosis of benign from malignant melanonychia, the ABCDEF rule was designed (Levit et al. 2000).

Dermatoscopy is a useful adjunct to the clinical diagnosis (Braun et al. 2007). A gray background and thin gray lines were associated with melanocyte activation, ethnic and drug-induced pigmentation, and a brown background and regular brown lines were linked with nevus, whereas melanoma shows a brown background and irregular brown lines (Ronger et al. 2002). A recent study showed that longitudinal melanonychia in individuals with skin phototypes IV, V, and VI often shows a brown or even black background, despite being only functional hypermelanosis (Astur Mde et al. 2016). However, both in children as well as in congenital nevi, irregularities may be seen that are commonly observed in adults with subungual melanoma. (Di Chiacchio et al. 2013; Goldminz et al. 2013). Direct matrix inspection (Fig. 6.6a–c) and matrix dermatoscopy reliably differentiate lentigines and nevi from melanoma (Hirata et al. 2005, 2006, 2011).

In a study of 137 cases of longitudinal melanonychia, 72 were considered type I owing to functional melanocyte activation, lentigo, and nevus; they did not show enlargement during a follow-up of a mean of 5 years. Fifty-two were classified as type II melanonychia and five of them demonstrated enlargement during follow-up; they were biopsied and three showed lentigo or nevus whereas two were in situ melanomas. The remaining 13 brown bands were classified as type III melanonychia and histologically diagnosed as melanoma in situ (Sawada et al. 2014).

The diagnostic gold standard is histopathological examination of an adequate biopsy specimen, ideally an excisional biopsy. Depending on the width of the melanonychia, different techniques such as punch, fusiform, crescentic, or lateral longitudinal biopsies are available. The superficial tangential biopsy allows large areas of the matrix to be biopsied, virtually without the risk of post-biopsy nail dystrophy (Haneke 1999). A quantitative study of the density of melanocytes yielded a mean melanocyte count of 15.3, a median of 14, and a range of 5–31 per millimeter stretch of the basal layer in lentigo contrast to mean and median counts of 7.7 and 7.5, range 4–9 for controls and a much higher number for invasive (102 and 92.5, range 52–212) and in situ melanoma (58.9 and 51, range 39–156) respectively (Amin et al. 2008). However, we have seen higher numbers of melanocytes per millimeter stretch of the basal layer of the matrix epithelium in many cases (Fig. 6.7).

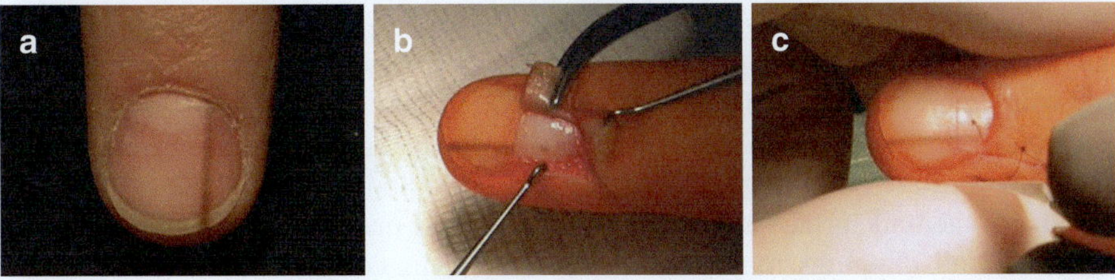

Fig. 6.6 Lentigo of the matrix. (**a**) Clinical photograph. (**b**) Lentigo of the matrix seen as a brown oval lesion. (**c**) After tangential excision, the nail plate has been laid back and stitched in place

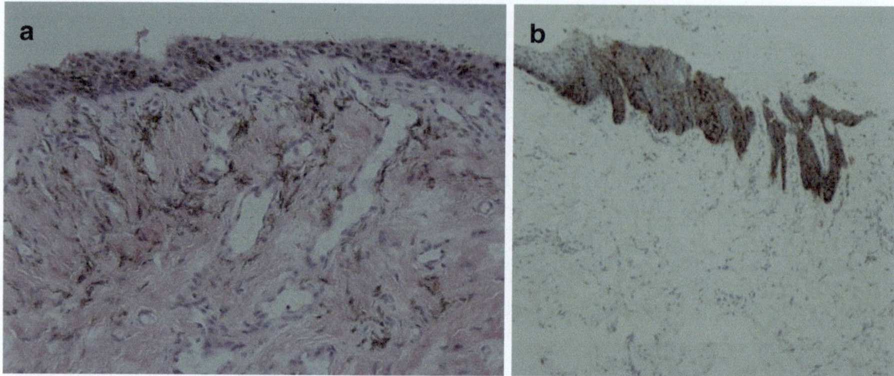

Fig. 6.7 Histology of a matrix lentigo with many melanocytes and huge masses of melanophages. (**a**) Hematoxylin and eosin-stained section of a tangential excision specimen showing an increased number of melanocytes in the matrix epithelium and melanophages in the dermis. (**b**) MelanA staining demonstrates a tremendous increase in the number of active melanocytes, but the melanophages are not stained

To differentiate subungual nevi from melanoma, DNA ploidy investigations were used (Asahina et al. 1993). Multiple gene amplifications are found in subungual melanomas early in their progression, about one-half of them in the cyclin D1 locus (Bastian 2003). Comparative genomic hybridization also allowed the diagnosis of a subungual melanoma to be made in a 13-year-old girl (Takata et al. 2003).

Differential Diagnosis

The clinical differential diagnosis of lentigines and nevi comprises virtually all melanocytic processes, such as functional melanonychia and melanoma, inflammatory nail diseases in darker pigmented individuals, hormonal diseases such as Addison and Nelson syndrome (Chang et al. 2013), many drugs, epithelial tumors with melanocyte population, such as pigmented Bowen disease, onychopapilloma (Fig. 6.8), onychomatricoma (Fig. 6.9), subungual hematoma (Fig. 6.10), infections with chromogenic bacteria such as pigmentation due to *Proteus* spp., *Klebsiella* spp. (Fig. 6.11) and *Pseudomonas aeruginosa*, fungal melanonychia from *Trichophyton rubrum* var. *nigricans* (Fig. 6.12) and a variety of molds (Fig. 6.13), exogenous nail pigmentation due to silver nitrate (Fig. 6.14), dirt, tar, ornamental stains (Fig. 6.15), heavy smoking and many more. Fumagoid bodies (Medlar bodies) were once seen to cause longitudinal melanonychia (Ko et al. 2005). Except for the melanocytic processes, the other pigmentations are not fine granular and argentaffin. Staining from enterobacteria is usually on the nail surface and can be scraped off, as many other exogenous discolorations. Nail clippings may contain nests of nevus cells, but intraungual single melanocytes are considered to be melanoma cells.

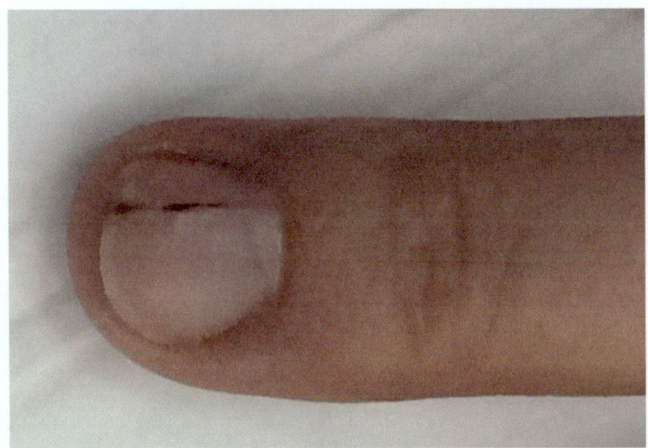

Fig. 6.8 Onychopapilloma with dark splinter hemorrhages

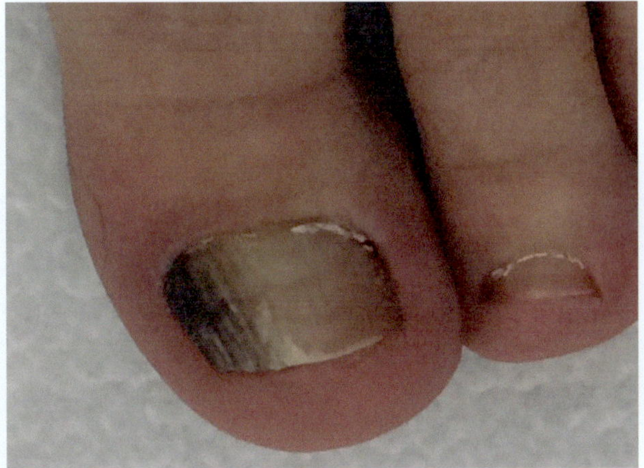

Fig. 6.9 Pigmented onychomatricoma of the big toe in a 51-year-old woman

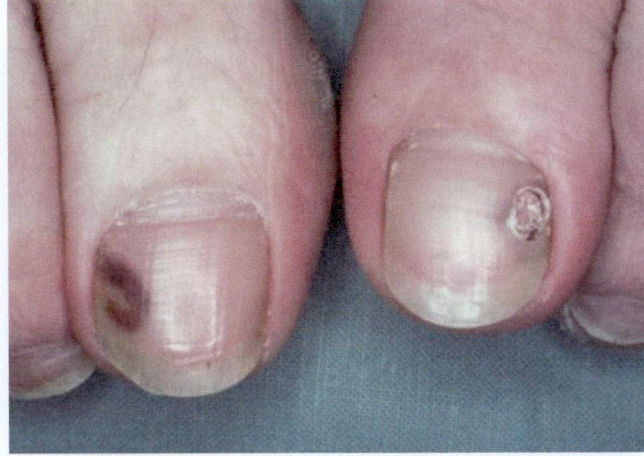

Fig. 6.10 Subungual hematoma due to friction. A disc of nail of the left big toenail has been punched out for the diagnosis of blood accumulation using the benzidine test

Fig. 6.11 Bacterial stain due to enterobacteria

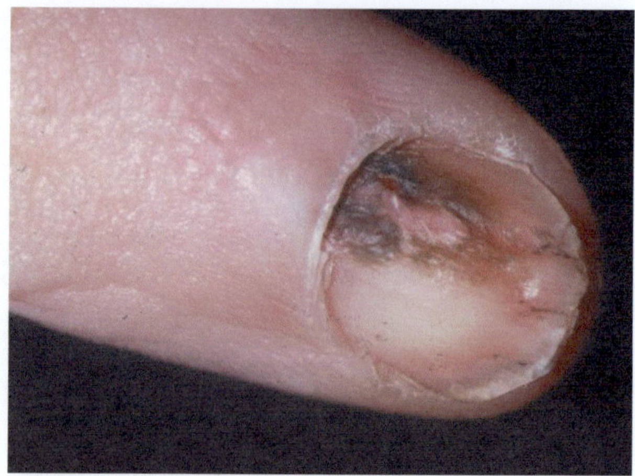

Fig. 6.12 Post-traumatic single-digit black onychomycosis due to *Trichophyton rubrum* in a 34-year-old black cook

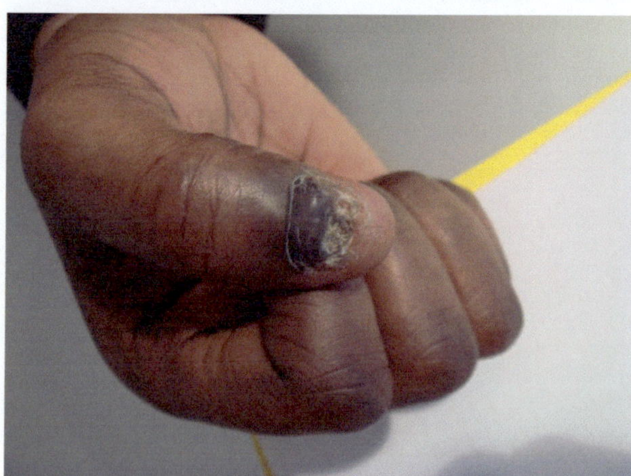

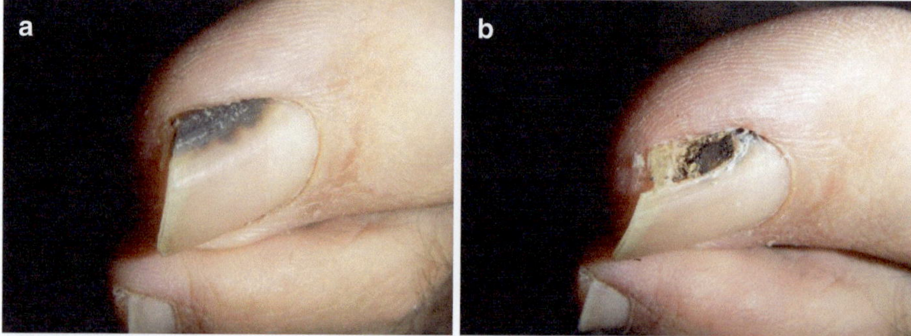

Fig. 6.13 Black onychomycosis due to molds (**a**) Clinical photograph (**b**) The nail plate has been partially cut away over the pigmentation revealing a jet-black keratotic mass

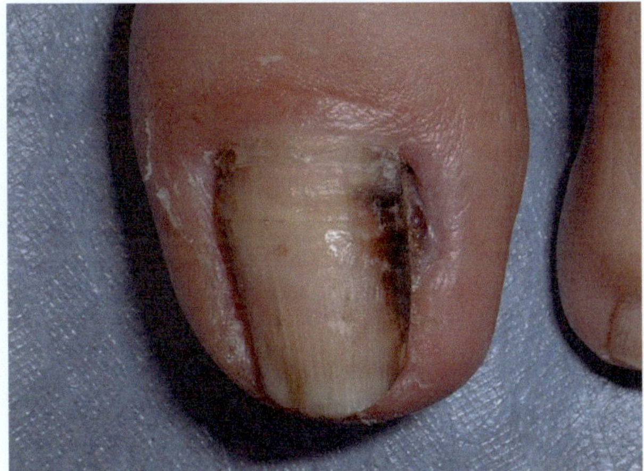

Fig. 6.14 Silver nitrate stain of the lateral nail margin due to therapeutic etching of granulation tissue

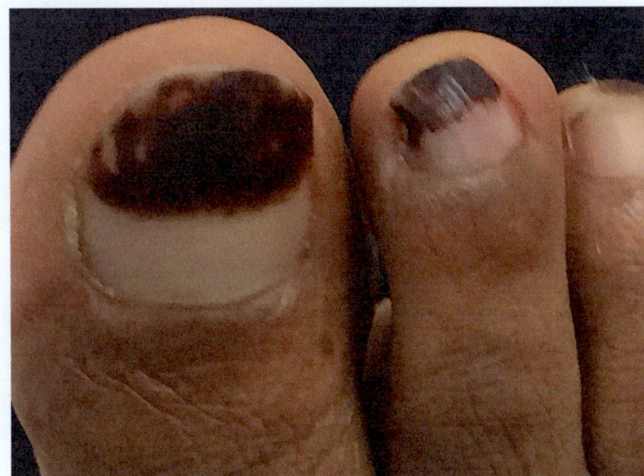

Fig. 6.15 Toenails of a 34-year-old black woman with a dark stain due to p-phenylene diamine adulterated henna applied for ornamental reasons. The staining grows out with its proximal margin being parallel to the free margin of the nail fold, which is proof of the exogenous nature of the dark nail stain

Treatment of Nail Lentigo and Nevi

Although it is our policy to remove acquired lentigines and nevi of the nail whenever the patient or his parents want this, many authors try to avoid surgery and rely instead on conservative diagnostic measures such as dermatoscopy or laser scanning microscopy. This may be correct for many cases, particularly in children; however, over a period of more than 30 years the number of invasive thick ungual melanomas that we have seen has dramatically decreased, and we believe that early excision of suspicious lesions is the right way to avoid thick melanomas (Haneke 2012). For lentigines and acquired nevi, which are almost invariably junctional and very rarely compound nevi, the diagnostic tangential excision is usually sufficient and therapeutic (Fig. 6.6). Even when a light brown streak re-occurs the histopathological diagnosis is made with certainty.

Outlook: Future Developments

Although quite common, particularly in more deeply pigmented individuals, melanonychias are still often overlooked or incorrectly diagnosed. It is not rare that a patient presents to his family physician for years or decades with a brown nail streak that gradually increases in color intensity and widens – unmistakable signs of proliferation and in most cases of malignancy. It is not the lack of examination tools, but rather the lack of awareness of potential malignant development that ungual melanomas are often not diagnosed or diagnosed too late. Certainly, more precise criteria for the diagnosis of matrix lentigines and nevi will be developed and refinement of confocal laser scanning microscopy criteria will enable us to differentiate, at least in many cases, lentigines from nevi, and above all from subungual melanoma.

> **Summary for the Clinician**
> Lentigines and nevi of the nail matrix are often the cause of a brown longitudinal band in the nail plate. Whereas such bands are usually benign in children, they should raise suspicion when they develop in adults over 30–40 years of age.

References

Agusti-Mejias A, Messeguer F, Febrer I, Alegre V. Congenital subungual and periungual melanocytic nevus. Acta Dermosifliograf. 2013;104:446–8.

Amin B, Nehal KS, Jungbluth AA, Zaidi B, Brady MS, Coit DC, Zhou Q, Busam KJ. Histologic distinction between subungual lentigo and melanoma. Am J Surg Pathol. 2008;32:835–43.

Asahina A, Matsuyama T, Tsuchida T, Nakagawa H, Seki T, Otsuka F, Ishibashi Y. Two cases of infantile subungual pigmented nevi with Hutchinson's sign. Nihon Hifuka Gakkai Zasshi. 1989;99:899–906.

Asahina A, Chi HI, Otsuka F. Subungual pigmented nevus: evaluation of DNA ploidy in six cases. J Dermatol. 1993;20:466–72.

Astur Mde M, Farkas CB, Junqueira JP, Enokihara MM, Enokihara MY, Michalany N, Hirata SH. Reassessing melanonychia striata in phototypes IV, V, and VI patients. Dermatol Surg. 2016;42:183–90.

Bastian BC. Understanding the progression of melanocytic neoplasia using genomic analysis: from fields to cancer. Oncogene. 2003;22:3081–6.

Braun RP, Baran R, Le Gal FA, Dalle S, Ronger S, Pandolfi R, Gaide O, French LE, Laugier P, Saurat JH, Marghoob AA, Thomas L. Diagnosis and management of nail pigmentations. J Am Acad Dermatol. 2007;56:835–47.

Causeret AS, Skowron F, Viallard AM, Balme B, Thomas L. Subungual blue nevus. J Am Acad Dermatol. 2003;49:310–2.

Chang P, Román V, Monterroso MA, Castro Benincasa ML, Cordonón C, Rivera S. Síndrome de Nelson. Dermatol Cosm Med Quir. 2013;11:199–202.

Coskey RJ, Magnel TD, Bernacki EG. Congenital subungual nevus. J Am Acad Dermatol. 1983;9:747–51.

Di Chiacchio N, Cadore De Farias D, Piraccini BM, Hirata SH, Richert B, Zaiac M, Daniel R, Fanti PA, Andre J, Ruben BS, Fleckman P, Rich P, Haneke E, Chang P, Cherit JD, Scher R,

Tosti A. Consenso sobre dermatoscopia da placa ungueal em melanoníquias. Consensus on melanonychia nail plate dermoscopy. An Bras Dermatol. 2013;88:313–7.

Goettmann-Bonvallot S, André J, Belaich S. Longitudinal melanonychia in children: a clinical and histopathologic study of 40 cases. J Am Acad Dermatol. 1999;41:17–22.

Goldminz AM, Wolpowitz D, Gottlieb AB, Krathen MS. Congenital subungual melanocytic nevus with a pseudo-Hutchinson sign. Dermatol Online J. 2013;19(4):8.

Haneke E. Laugier-Hunziker-Baran-Syndrom. Hautarzt. 1991;42:512–5.

Haneke E. Operative Therapie akraler und subungualer Melanome. In: Rompel R, Petres J, editors. Operative und onkologische Dermatologie, Fortschritte der operativen und onkologischen Dermatologie, vol. 15. Berlin: Springer; 1999. p. 210–4.

Haneke E. Ungual melanoma – controversies in diagnosis and treatment. Dermatol Ther. 2012;25:510–24.

Hirata SH, Yamada S, Almeida FA, Tomomori-Yamashita J, Enokihara MY, Paschoal FM, Enokihara MM, Outi CM, Michalany NS. Dermoscopy of the nail bed and matrix to assess melanonychia striata. J Am Acad Dermatol. 2005;53:884–6.

Hirata SH, Yamada S, Almeida FA, Enokihara MY, Rosa IP, Enokihara MM, Michalany NS. Dermoscopic examination of the nail bed and matrix. Int J Dermatol. 2006;45:28–30.

Hirata SH, Yamada S, Enokihara MY, Di Chiacchio N, de Almeida FA, Enokihara MM, Michalany NS, Zaiac M, Tosti A. Patterns of nail matrix and bed of longitudinal melanonychia by intraoperative dermatoscopy. J Am Acad Dermatol. 2011;65:297–303.

Kawabata Y, Ohara K, Hino H, Tamaki K. Two kinds of Hutchinson's sign, benign and malignant. J Am Acad Dermatol. 2001;44:305–7.

Ko CJ, Sarantopoulos GP, Pai G, Binder SW. Longitudinal melanonychia of the toenails with presence of Medlar bodies on biopsy. J Cutan Pathol. 2005;32:63–5.

Kopf AW, Waldo E. Melanonychia striata. Aust J Dermatol. 1980;21:59–70.

Léauté-Labrèze C, Biouliac-Sage P, Taïeb A. Longitudinal melanonychia in children. Arch Dermatol. 1996;132:167–9.

Leung AK, Woo TY. A subungual nevus in a Filipino child. Pediatr Dermatol. 2004;21:462–5.

Levit EK, Kagen MH, Scher RK, Grossman M, Altman E. The ABC rule for clinical detection of subungual melanoma. J Am Acad Dermatol. 2000;42:269–74.

Libow LF, Casey TJ, Varela CD. Congenital subungual nevus in a black infant. Cutis. 1995;56:154–6.

Makhoul EN, Ayoub NM, Helou JF, Abadjian GA. Familial Laugier-Hunziker syndrome. J Am Acad Dermatol. 2003;49:S143–5.

Moore RT, Chae KA, Rhodes AR. Laugier and Hunziker pigmentation: a lentiginous proliferation of melanocytes. J Am Acad Dermatol. 2004;50:S70–4.

Ohtsuka H, Hori Y, Ando M. Nevus of the little finger with a remarkable nail deformity. Plast Reconstr Surg. 1978;61:108–11.

Pomerance J, Kopf AW, Ramos L, Waldo E, Grossman JA. A large, pigmented nail bed lesion in a child. Ann Plast Surg. 1994;33:80–2.

Ronger S, Touzet S, Ligeron C, Balme B, Viallard AM, Barrut D, Colin C, Thomas L. Dermoscopic examination of nail pigmentation. Arch Dermatol. 2002;138:1327–33.

Rosendahl C, Cameron A, Wilkinson D, Belt P, Williamson R, Weedon D. Nail matrix melanoma: consecutive cases in a general practice. Dermatol Pract Concept. 2012;2(2):202a13.

Sawada M, Yokota K, Matsumoto T, Shibata S, Yasue S, Sakakibara A, Kono M, Akiyama M. Proposed classification of longitudinal melanonychia based on clinical and dermoscopic criteria. Int J Dermatol. 2014;53:581–5.

Shukla VK, Hughes LE. How common are benign subungual naevi? Eur J Surg Oncol. 1992;18:249–50.

Takata M, Maruo K, Kageshita T, Ikeda S, Ono T, Shirasaki F, Takehara K, Bastian BC. Two cases of unusual acral melanocytic tumors: illustration of molecular cytogenetics as a diagnostic tool. Hum Pathol. 2003;34:89–92.

Theunis A, Richert B, Sass U, Lateur N, Sales F, André J. Immunohistochemical study of 40 cases of longitudinal melanonychia. Am J Dermatopathol. 2011;33:27–34.

Tomizawa K. Early malignant melanoma manifested as longitudinal melanonychia: subungual melanoma may arise from suprabasal melanocytes. Br J Dermatol. 2000;143:431–4.

Tosti A, Baran R, Piraccini BM, et al. Nail matrix nevi: a clinical and histopathologic study of twenty-two patients. J Am Acad Dermatol. 1996;34:765–71.

Tosti A, Piraccini BM, Baran R. The melanocyte system of the nails and its disorders. In: Nordlund JJ, Boissy RE, Hearing VJ, King R, Ortonne JP, editors. The Pigmentary System. New York: Oxford University Press; 1998. p. 937–42.

Valero A, Sherf K. Pigmented nails in Peutz-Jeghers syndrome. Am J Gastroenterol. 1965;43:56–9.

Vidal S, Sanz A, Hernández B, Sánchez Yus E, Requena L, Baran R. Subungual blue naevus. Br J Dermatol. 1997;137:1023–5.

Subungual Melanoma

7

Judith Domínguez-Cherit, Daniela Gutiérrez-Mendoza,
Mariana de Anda-Juarez, Verónica Fonte-Avalos,
and Sonia Toussaint- Caire

Key Features
- Longitudinal melanonychia is the first sign of subungual melanoma.
- Subungual melanoma (SUM) is a type of acral lentiginous melanoma (ALM) that is uncommon in fair-skinned individuals (0.7–3.5%) (Sureda et al. 2011).
- SUM is more frequent in patients with darker skin phototypes III–VI, such as Hispanics, Asians, and African–Americans, accounting for up to 20% of all cutaneous melanomas (Dominguez-Cherit et al. 2008; Phan et al. 2006).
- The horizontal or radial growth phase is very slow, but when vertical growth is present the prognosis of SUM, compared with other types of melanomas, is the poorest.
- When melanoma in situ is diagnosed, conservative treatment is an option.

Introduction

Subungual melanoma (SUM) is a variant of acral lentiginous melanoma (ALM), and nearly all cases arise from nail matrix melanocytes.

Patients commonly report trauma as a related factor preceding the diagnosis of melanonychia and melanoma; however, its exact role in the pathogenesis of the disease has not been established (Briggs 1984; Mohrle and Hafner 2002).

J. Domínguez-Cherit (✉)
Instituto Nacional de Ciencias Médicas y Nutrición Salvador Zubiran, Mexico City, Mexico
e-mail: judom59@hotmail.com

D. Gutiérrez-Mendoza • M. de Anda-Juarez • V. Fonte-Avalos • S. Toussaint-Caire
Hospital General " Dr Manuel Gea Gonzalez", México City, México

© Springer International Publishing Switzerland 2017
N. Di Chiacchio, A. Tosti (eds.), *Melanonychias*,
DOI 10.1007/978-3-319-44993-7_7

The frequency of racial melanonychia in dark-skinned patients is high, occurring in 68% of Hispanics with longitudinal melanonychia (LM). In a study of 68 patients with LM, only 2% had a diagnosis of melanoma (Dominguez-Cherit et al. 2008). For this reason, it is easy to minimize the appearance of melanonychia in this population, thus making the diagnosis of SUM difficult in the early phases. However, in those with darker skin, (phototypes III–VI), SUM is not rare, corresponding to 20% of all types of melanoma and 50% of ALMs (Herrera and Aco 2010; De la Fuente and Ocampo 2010).

Epidemiology

SUM is uncommon in fair-skinned individuals. At the University of Tübingen, a dermatological unit dedicated to the study and treatment of melanoma found that the incidence ranges from 0.7% to 7% (Kuchelmeister et al. 2000). In a study conducted over 11 years at this center, a total of 112 cases of ALM were reported. Only 19 cases of subungual melanoma occurred in the oldest age group. Interestingly, the prognosis of these patients was poor, similar to those with nodular melanoma. In Japan, Takematsu et al. (1985) found that 19% of SUM cases appeared on the fingers. In Mexico, per the National Cancer Institute, 31% of melanomas were of the acral lentiginous type, and SUM accounted for almost half of these cases (Herrera and Aco 2010; De la Fuente and Ocampo 2010). The statistics were higher in a dermatology department of a general hospital in Mexico City: of the total 165 patients with melanoma, 43% presented with ALM, and 36% of these were SUM (Káram-Orantes et al. 2008).

History

In 1886, Hutchinson described melanomas of the nail bed, or melanotic whitlow (Hutchinson 1886). In 1934, Boyer introduced the term acral melanoma. In 1972, Luprescu reported that the histology of this type of melanoma was like a lentigo maligna and in 1976, Reed described it as a distinct histopathological subtype (Luprescu et al. 1973; Reed 1976).

Recently, acral cutaneous melanoma has been considered to have histopathological characteristics of superficial spreading melanoma (30%), acral lentiginous melanoma (60%), or nodular melanoma (9%) (Kuchelmeister et al. 2000) depending on the anatomical site of presentation.

Clinical Features

Melanonychia Characteristics

Width

The main presentation is LM that can vary in width. It may start as a narrow band of pigmentation and progressively cover the whole nail plate (total melanonychia) (Fig. 7.1).

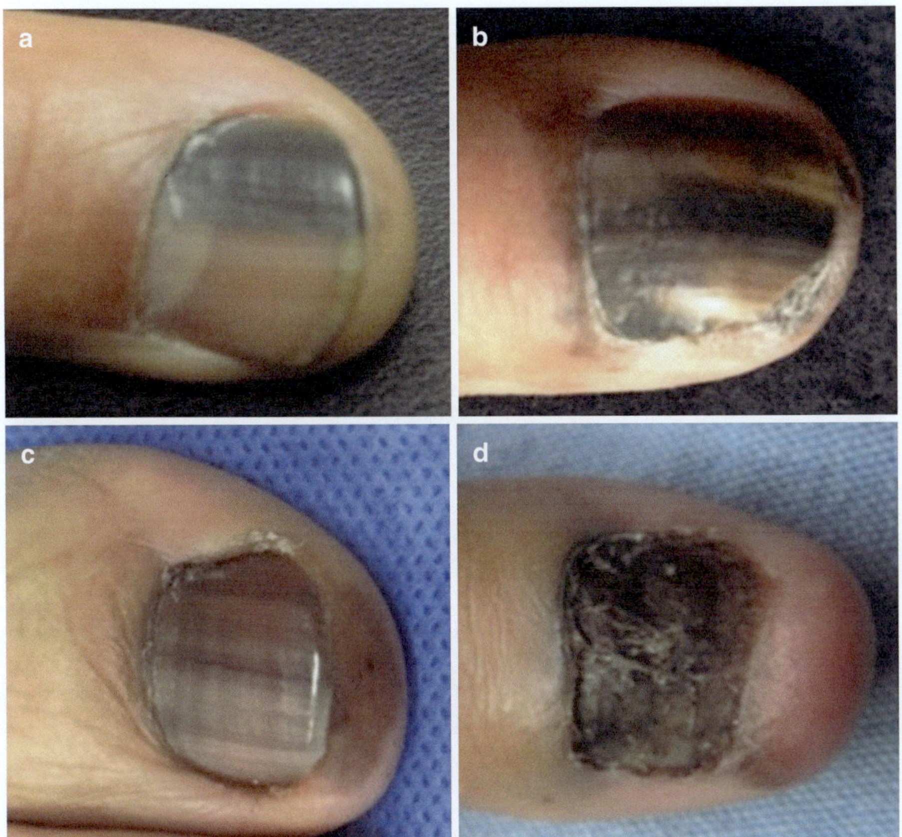

Fig. 7.1 Longitudinal melanonychia progression. (**a**) Subungual melanoma can present as a homogeneous *black longitudinal band*, or it may progress slowly to total melanonychia. (**b**) Heterogeneous black pigmentation affects more than half of the nail plate. (**c**) Total melanonychia with multiple *light brown* irregular bands of heterogeneous spacing and width. (**d**) It is not uncommon to observe dystrophy of the nail plate in advanced cases. Note the variation in colors, ranging from light brown to black and the presence of Hutchinson's sign in the four cases

The width of the melanonychia is an important marker of melanoma. According to a study in Hispanics, a band measuring 4–6 mm resulted in a diagnosis of melanoma in 1 case, and 2 cases of those had total melanonychia (Dominguez-Cherit et al. 2008).

Shape
It is characteristic to see a longitudinal pigmented band of pyramidal or triangular shape, with the widest part near the cuticle, meaning that there is progressive growth (Fig. 7.2).

Color
Melanonychia can range from light brown to black, red, or a mixture of colors. Color is a poor marker for melanoma; however, variegation can help to distinguish

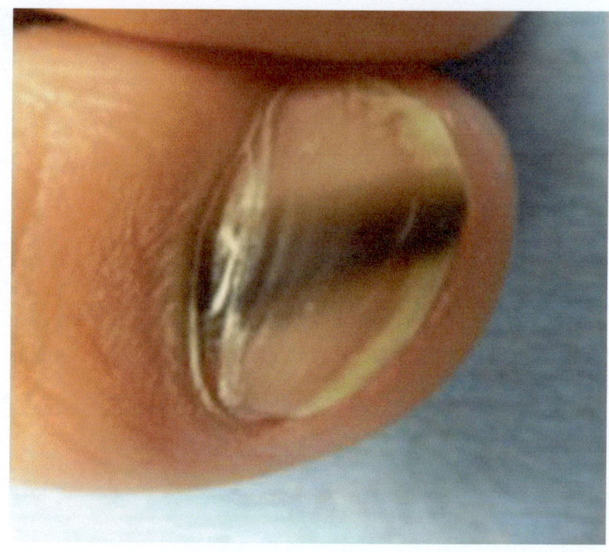

Fig. 7.2 Longitudinal melanonychia with a pyramidal shape. A medial longitudinal band with proximal widening and distal tapering can be observed. Note the variegated color, width, and blurred edges of the pigmented band

between benign and malignant causes, especially when other signs such as width or progression of melanonychia are present. With a dermoscope, visualization of gray, red or brown color can determine the cause of the melanonychia and other diagnoses such as subungual hematoma or drug-induced melanonychia can be ruled out (see section "Dermoscopy") (Fig. 7.1).

Location

Subungual melanoma is more common in the fingernails. Seventy-five percent of SUM cases are localized to the first and middle fingers (De Anda Juárez et al. 2016).

History

In children, it is important to consider whether LM has been present since infancy, but not changed in color or size. If so, it should be considered a nevus, but in an LM in a child or a young adult that has been growing and presenting color variegation from light brown to dark brown, an early SUM should be suspected.

Other Findings

When nail dystrophy is present, especially changes in the texture of the nail plate that can range from minimal to complete destruction of the nail surface, invasive SUM should be considered (Figs. 7.1d and 7.3). If pigmentation extends to the hyponychium or is evident in the eponychium, this is considered a Hutchinson sign (Fig. 7.1). In most cases, it is asymptomatic, but in the invasive phase it could be

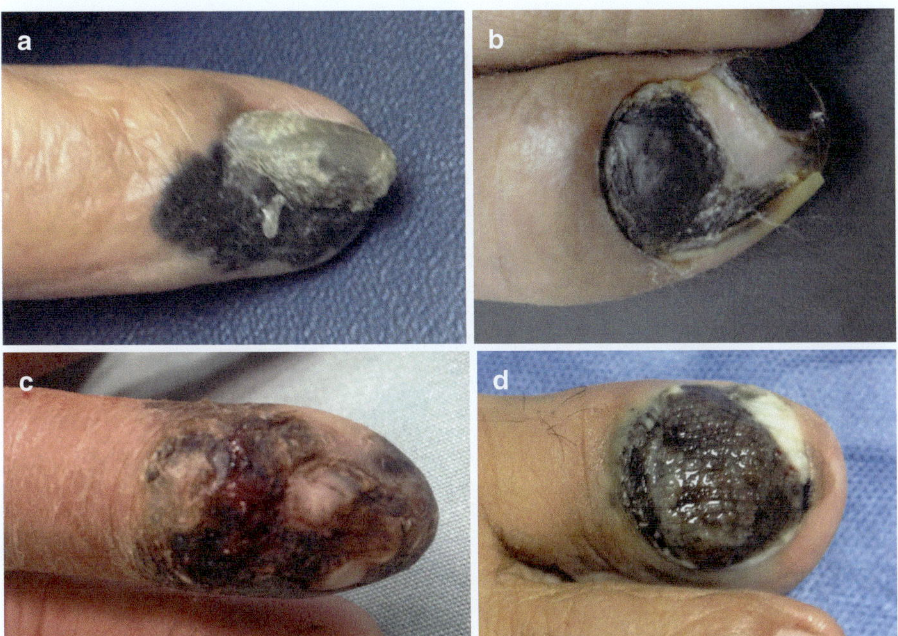

Fig. 7.3 Invasive subungual melanoma with dystrophy. All cases show signs of disease progression: partial or total nail plate destruction, ulceration, nodule formation, and Hutchinson's sign

painful, bleeding occurs, and secondary infection could be present (Phan et al. 2006; De Anda Juárez et al. 2016).

Certain protein-decoder genes controlling the cellular cycle have been described, as a special feature of this type of melanoma. One of the most important of these is CDKN2A, also known as INK4a. It is located in chromosome 9p21 and codifies for the p16 protein, which is an important negative regulator of the cell cycle. Sixty-seven percent of ALM cases are known to have a low or null function of p16. Melanoma with this characteristic finding correlates with more aggressive conduct and a bad prognosis compared with other variants of melanoma (Bastian et al. 2000; Chana et al. 2000).

Diagnostic Clues

There are no definitive clinical criteria to diagnose SUM in an early phase and all cases must be individualized; however, clues to aid in the diagnosis are summarized in Table 7.1.

Table 7.1 Diagnostic clues in subungual melanoma

	High degree of suspicion	Low degree of suspicion	Tips
Age	40–60 years	Children	Do not rule out in children even though it is less common
Gender	F=M	F=M	
Race	African–Americans, Asians, and Hispanics	Caucasians	
Location	Hands	Toes	Thumb, index finger, and great toe most commonly affected, but can affect any finger
Number of fingers	Single nail	Multiple nails	When there is racial melanonychia, more than one finger may be affected
Melanonychia characteristics			
Width	4–6 mm or total width melanonychia	Less than 4 mm	Lines must be regular in width, shape, and spacing
Progression	Growing	Stable	
Shape	Wider at the proximal nail fold (growing neoplasm)	Regular shape	
Lines	Regular	Irregular	
Space	Regular	Irregular	
Colors	Variegation, (multiple colors)	One color	In onychomycosis color variegation and dystrophy are not uncommon
Dystrophy[a]	Present	Absent	
Other findings[a]	Hutchinson's sign	Absent	
	Ulceration		
	Bleeding		

[a]Risk factors for invasive melanoma

Dermoscopy

Dermoscopy is a non-invasive method that helps to differentiate the distinct causes of melanonychia. It can be performed with or without polarized light. The latter requires the use of gel for better visualization (Dominguez-Cherit et al. 2010).

In melanonychia, owing to the increased number of melanocytes, as in the case of a nevus or melanoma, a brown background pigment is observed (Fig. 7.4a). Furthermore, in addition to this background color, in subungual melanoma, a pattern of heterogeneous longitudinal brown or black lines can be seen. The bands have irregular thickness and spacing and lose their parallelism (Figs. 7.4b, and 7.5). Pigment granules can also be found. Micro-Hutchinson's sign refers to cuticle pigmentation that is evident only thorough a dermoscope, but is not visible to the naked eye. Signs of melanoma are irregular brown melanonychia, together with nail plate dystrophy, and a triangular shape of the longitudinal band that indicates the radial expansion of the melanoma (Fig. 7.5) (Di Chiacchio et al. 2013).

Fig. 7.4 (**a**) Dermoscopy of *light brown* longitudinal background pigmentation. This example may corre spond to melanonychia due to an increase in the number of melanocytes as in nevus or melanoma. (**b**) Dermoscopy of a band with a *light brown* background and irregular lines that lose their parallelism. This type of melanonychia with irregular color, width, and spacing corresponds to melanoma

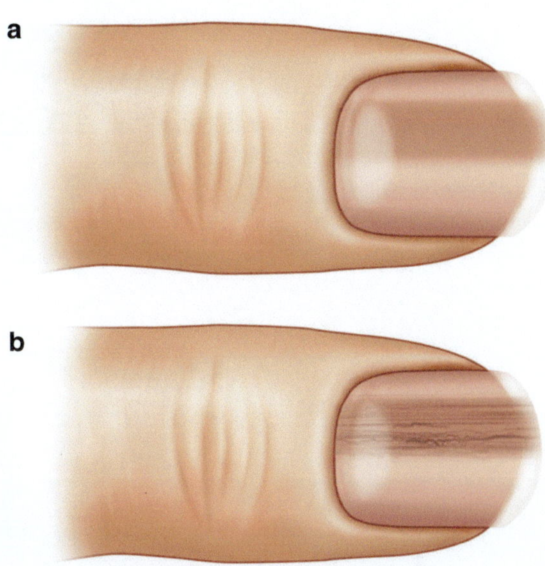

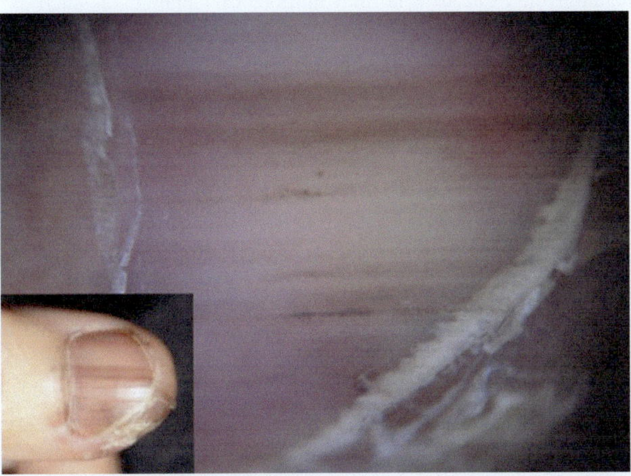

Fig. 7.5 Dermoscopy of a subungual melanoma. Clinical photograph of *light brown*, subtle total melanonychia of the right thumb. Dermoscopy shows *brown* background pigmentation with irregularity in color, width, and spacing. Note that the melanonychia covers the totality of the nail plate surface; there are irregular globules and Hutchinson's and micro-Hutchinson's sign

Gray background color (melanonychia without an increase in the number of melanocytes, but with melanin deposits, as in drug-induced lesions) and a red pattern (as melanonychia due to hematoma) are important patterns in the differential diagnosis of melanoma (Fig. 7.6) (Dominguez-Cherit et al. 2010).

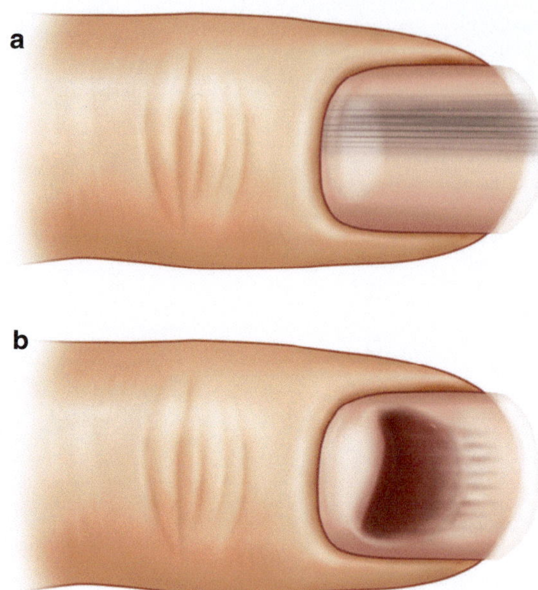

Fig. 7.6 (**a**) Dermoscopy with a *light gray* background color and parallel lines. This example may correspond to melanonychia due to a normal number of melanocytes such as in drug-induced melanonychia or racial pigmentation. (**b**) Dermoscopy shows a red blotch or globules with distal filamentous lines. This example may correspond to subungual hematoma, an important differential diagnosis of subungual melanoma

It is also possible to perform intraoperative dermoscopy with polarized light. This procedure helps in the evaluation of the thickness, spacing, and color of the band. Irregular morphology in the lines and the presence of globules indicate unequivocal melanoma of the nail matrix. It is also useful for evaluating the best place to perform a biopsy (Di Chiacchio et al. 2013).

Biopsy

Biopsy of SUM must include the nail matrix, as it helps in the diagnosis, classification, prognosis, and treatment of melanoma. The type of biopsy that is performed depends on the ability of the surgeon and the histopathologist, and a close relationship between them can increase the likelihood of successful results.

The localization of the melanonychia can also dictate the type of biopsy. In lateral melanonychia, a lateral longitudinal biopsy is the best option. It is one of the

Table 7.2 Types of biopsy for subungual melanoma

Type of melanonychia	Type of biopsy	Procedure
Lateral	Lateral longitudinal	Ellipse
Medial	Nail matrix	3-mm width punch/shave/tangential

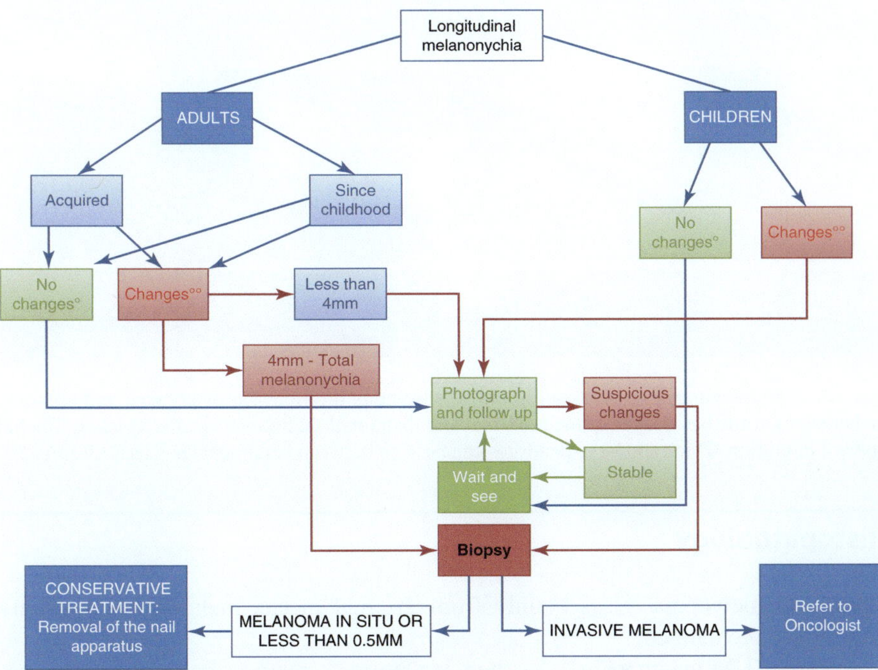

Fig. 7.7 Algorithmic approach to the diagnosis and treatment of melanonychia in children and adults. °No change refers to no difference in width, color or dystrophy of the nail plate. °°Change refers to any difference in width, color, or presence of dystrophy of the nail plate

most complete specimens as it includes cuticle, matrix, nail, nail bed, and hyponychium. In medial melanonychia a nail matrix biopsy can be performed. There are several techniques, which include a 3-mm punch, an elliptical biopsy, or a shave biopsy (Table 7.2).

Biopsy should be performed in all adult patients with acquired melanonychia who suffer progression regardless of the color or width of the band. In those with no changes or in children, a wait and see approach is suggested. Close examination with dermoscopy and photographs should be routine every 3–6 months and a biopsy must be performed if any change is detected (Fig. 7.7).

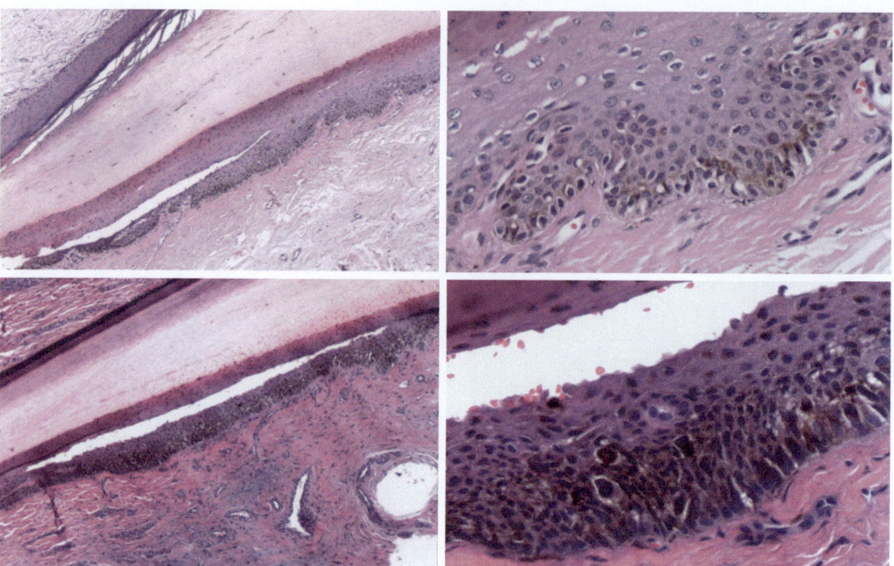

Fig. 7.8 Early subungual melanoma in situ. Lentiginous proliferation of atypical and enlarged melanocytes at the basal layer of the proximal and distal nail matrix with scattered intraepithelial upward migration. Thick and large dendrites can be seen between keratinocytes (H&E ×5 and ×20)

Histopathology

Subungual melanoma arises mainly from the nail matrix melanocytes and only rarely from the nailbed.

In early SUM in situ, (Fig. 7.8), there is a poorly circumscribed and uneven proliferation of atypical melanocytes along the basal layer, with a lentiginous growth pattern. The density of melanocytes per lineal millimeter of the epithelial–dermal junction is around 51, compared with 15 in subungual lentigos (Amin et al. 2008). Atypical melanocytes may have a dendritic, epithelioid or spindle appearance. They show hyperchromatic, pleomorphic, and enlarged nuclei (two to three times the size of basal keratinocyte nuclei), the presence of one or more prominent nucleoli, and expansion of the cytoplasm with fine melanin granules (Rhodes et al. 1989). Dendrites are thicker and larger, and may reach the highest epithelial layers.

In more advanced stages of SUM in situ (Fig. 7.9), there is confluence of atypical melanocytes along the basal layer of the nail matrix, formation of irregular nests, and haphazard pagetoid intraepithelial spread by more markedly atypical melanocytes. There is also a moderate to dense junctional and subjunctional inflammatory lymphocytic infiltrate. Melanocytic proliferation may extend to the nailbed epithelium, hyponychium, and eponychium (Hutchinson's sign), and melanin is distributed irregularly within the lesion.

Invasive SUM (Fig. 7.10), has a denser proliferation of markedly atypical melanocytes, arranged in larger aggregates and sheaths, and may lead to epithelial

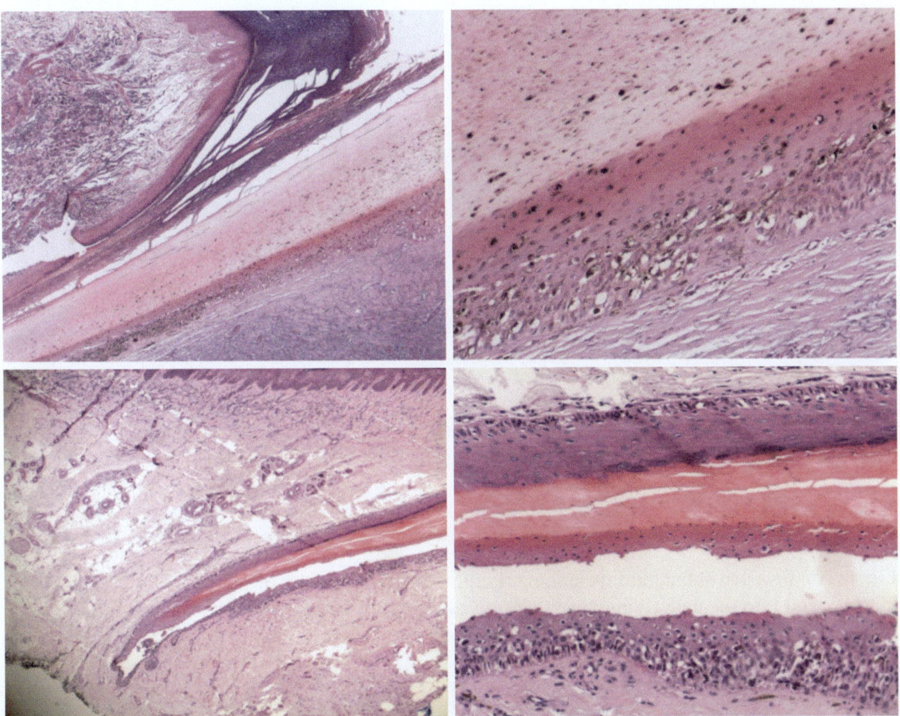

Fig. 7.9 Advanced subungual melanoma in situ. Denser and confluent proliferation of atypical melanocytes at the proximal and distal nail matrix extending into the epithelium of the proximal nailfold. There is marked pagetoid upward intraepithelial spread of melanocytes, which also show thick dendrites reaching the upper layers of the epithelium (H&E, ×5 and ×20)

consumption, nail dystrophy, and ulceration. The expanding tumor nests eventually destroy the nail apparatus and invade the onychodermis and adjacent acral skin.

Recognized histological features for prognosis are the same as in other cutaneous melanomas; however, some studies have not corroborated these outcome-predicting factors (Tan et al. 2007a). This is probably due to the difficulty of accurately measuring Clark's level and Breslow's thickness, because the distinction between papillary and reticular onychodermis is not clear, subcutaneous fat may be absent, and underlying bone is separated by only a thin dermal collagen layer.

Treatment

In situ, SUM should be treated with a wide 5-mm margin resection of nail apparatus (Fig. 7.7); the deep margin should reach the periosteum, with special care needed to remove the matrix horns completely (Fig. 7.11).

The treatment for invasive SUM is amputation of the distal phalanx.

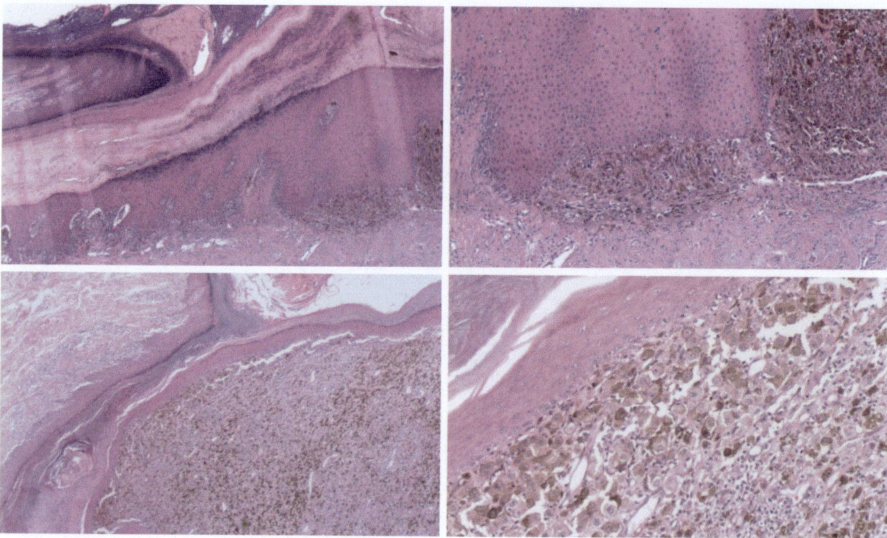

Fig. 7.10 Invasive subungual melanoma. Large nests and sheaths of markedly atypical melano-cytes extend into the underlying onychodermis altering the normal anatomy of the nail unit resulting in nail dystrophy (H&E, ×5 and ×20)

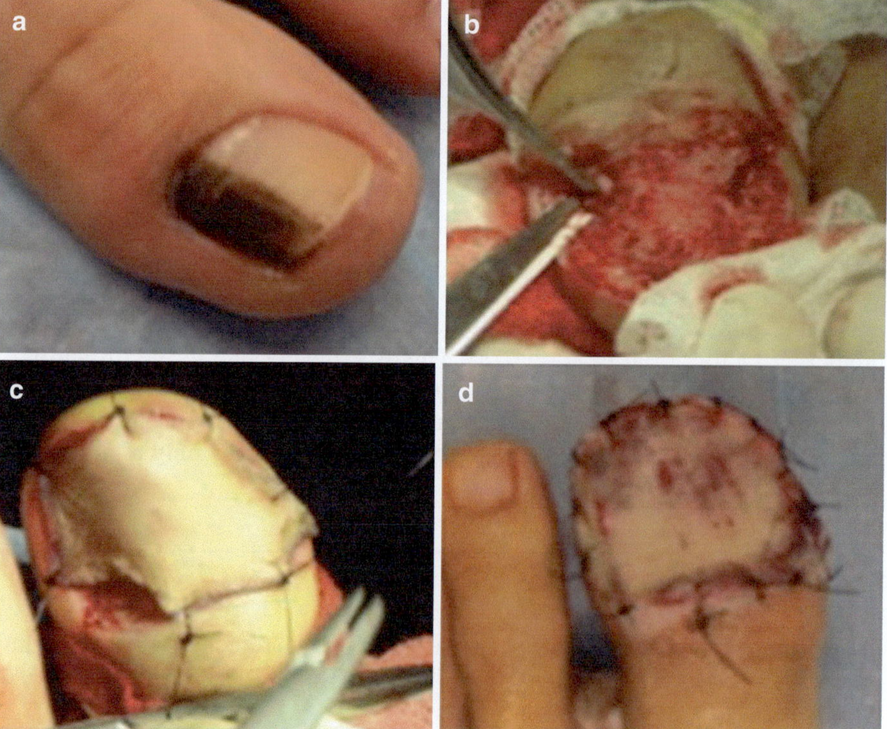

Fig. 7.11 Treatment of subungual melanoma. (**a**) Longitudinal melanonychia with diagnosis of subungual melanoma in situ. (**b**) Total excision of the nail apparatus. (**c**, **d**) A skin graft is used to close the wound

Sentinel lymph node biopsy should be performed in SUM >1 mm in depth and <1 mm with >1 mitosis per mm^2 or ulceration.

Studies have suggested that conservative surgical treatment for early SUM is justified, as the nail matrix area appears to be more resistant to invasion (Shin et al. 2014a, b).

> **Summary for the Clinician**
>
> Subungual melanoma is a variant of acral lentiginous melanoma, which is rare in Caucasians, but common in Asians, African—Americans, and Hispanics.
>
> Nail melanoma has a high mortality rate with a poor prognosis due to delayed diagnosis and invasive disease.
>
> In the early stages, it presents as a single nail longitudinal melanonychia 4–6 mm wide, with a proximal triangular shape. Color heterogeneity, blurred lateral borders, and Hutchinson's sign are very suggestive. With disease progression, the nail becomes dystrophic, with even complete destruction of the nail apparatus, or it presents as a pigmented or even amelanic bleeding tumor, which can be painful.
>
> The definitive diagnosis is made with a biopsy of the nail matrix. In situ, SUM should be treated with wide 5-mm margin resection of the nail apparatus. The treatment for invasive SUM is amputation of the distal phalanx.
>
> Sentinel lymph node biopsy should be performed in SUM >1 mm in depth and <1 mm with >1 mitosis per mm^2 or ulceration.
>
> Prognosis is directly related to the depth of invasion reported as Breslow's thickness in millimeters, which is why early detection and treatment are crucial for increasing survival (Mannava et al. 2013; Tan et al. 2007b; Cohen et al. 2008).

References

Amin B, et al. Histologic distinction between subungual lentigo and melanoma. Am J Surg Pathol. 2008;32:835–43.

Bastian B, Kashani S, Hamm H. Gene amplifications characterize acral melanoma and permit detection of occult timer cells in the surrounding skin. Cancer Reg. 2000;60:1968–73.

Briggs JC. The role of trauma in the etiology of malignant melanoma. Br J Plast Surg. 1984;37:514–6.

Chana JS, Grover R, Wilson GD. Analysis of p16 tumor suppressor gene expression in acral lentiginous melanoma. Br J Plast Surg. 2000;53:46–50.

Cohen T, Busam KJ, Patel A. Subungual melanoma: management considerations. Am J Surg. 2008;195:244–8.

De Anda Juárez M., Gutierrez-Mendoza D, Martínez Velasco A., Fonte Ávalos V., Martínez-Luna E, Toussaint-Caire S, Domínguez-Cherit J. Conservative surgical management of in-situ subungual melanoma. Long-term follow-up in Hispanic population An Bras Dermatol 91:846–848

De la Fuente A, Ocampo J. Melanoma cutáneo. Gac Med Mex. 2010;146:126–35.

Di Chiacchio N, Ruben B, Refkalevsky W, Loureiro M. Longitudinal Melanonychia. Clin Dermatol Nails Clin. 2013;31(5):594–601.

Dominguez-Cherit J, Roldan-Marin R, Pichardo-Velazquez P, Valente C, Fonte-Avalos V, Vega-Memije ME, Toussaint-Caire S. Melanocytic hyperplasia, and nail melanoma in a Hispanic population. J Am Acad Dermatol. 2008;59(5):785–91.

Dominguez-Cherit J, Fonte-Avalos V, Gutiérrez Mendoza D. Atlas de Uñas Elsevier, Mexico. 2010:31–6.

Herrera N, Aco A. El melanoma en México. Rev de especialidades médico-quirúrgicas. 2010;15(3):161–4.

Hutchinson J. Melanosis often non-black: melanotic whitlow. Br Med J. 1886;1:491.

Káram-Orantes M, Toussaint-Caire SJ, Veja-Memije E. Características clínicas e histopatológicas del melanoma maligno en el Hospital General "Dr. Manuel Gea González". Gac Méd Méx. 2008;144(3):219–23.

Kuchelmeister C, Schaumburg-Lever G, Garbe C. Acral cutaneous melanoma in caucasians: clinical features, histopathology and prognosis in 112 patients. Br J Dermatol. 2000;143(2):275–80.

Luprescu A, et al. Lentigo maligna of the fingertip; clinical, histologic and ultrastructural studies of two cases. Arch Dermatol. 1973;107:717–22.

Mannava K, Mannava S, Koman L, Robinson-Bostom L, Jellinek N. Longitudinal melanonychia: detection and management of nail melanoma. Hand Surg. 2013;18(1):133–9.

Mohrle M, Hafner HM. Is subungual melanoma related to trauma? Dermatology. 2002;204:259–61.

Phan A, Touzet S, Dalle S, Ronger-Savlé S, Balme B, Thomas L. Acral Lentiginous melanoma: a clinicoprognostic study of 126 cases. Br J Dermatol. 2006;155(3):561–9.

Reed RJ. Acral lentiginous melanoma. In: Hartman W, Kay S, Reed RJ, editors. New concepts in surgical pathology of the skin. New York: Wiley; 1976. p. 89–90.

Rhodes AR, Mihm MC, Weinstock MA. Dysplastic melanocytic nevi: a reproducible definition emphasizing cellular morphology. Mod Pathol. 1989;2:306–19.

Shin H-T, et al. Histopathological analysis of the progression pattern of subungual melanoma: late tendency of dermal invasion in the nail matrix area. Mod Pathol 2014a; 27:1461–1467.

Shin H-T, et al. A case of subungual melanoma with tumor invasion sparing the nail matrix dermis. Ann Dermatol. 2014b;26(5):655–6.

Sureda N, Phan A, Poulalhon N, Balme B, Dalle S, Thomas L. Conservative surgical management of subungual (matrix derived) melanoma: report of seven cases and literature review. Br J Dermatol. 2011;165(4):852–8.

Takematsu H, Obata M, Tomita Y, Kato T, Takahashi M, Abe R. Subungual melanoma. A clinico-pathologic study of 16 Japanese cases. Cancer. 1985;55(11):2725–31.

Tan K-B, et al. Subungual melanoma. A study of 124 cases highlighting features of early lesions, potential pitfalls in diagnosis, and guidelines for histologic reporting. J Surg Pathol. 2007a;31:1902–12.

Tan KB, Moncrieff M, Thompson JF. Subungual melanoma. A study of 124 cases highlighting features of early lesions, potential pitfalls in diagnosis, and guidelines for histologic reporting. Am J Surg Pathol. 2007b;31(12):1902–12.

Melanonychia in Children

8

B.M. Piraccini, Aurora Alessandrini, Emi Dika, and M. Starace

---

Key Features
- Melanonychia in children is usually due a nail matrix nevus.
- Nail melanoma in children is rare, and is exceptional in Caucasians.
- Clinical and dermoscopic parameters used in adults are not valid in children.
- Criteria suggesting biopsy are rapid growth and black color.
- Melanonychia in children requires only follow-up over time.

Introduction

Melanonychia in children is less common than in adults and it is different with regard to incidence and clinical and dermoscopic features. Today, melanonychia in children needs standardized management. Almost all cases of longitudinal melanonychia (LM) in children are benign; most are due to melanocytic nevi or lentigos affecting the nail matrix. Nail melanoma in children is extremely rare. Moreover, the prevalence of nail melanoma in children is extremely variable depending on their race and is more common in pigmented races. The need for biopsy in childhood melanonychia is more frequently discussed and less definite than in adults because LM in children often shows often frightening signs, mimicking aspects of nail melanoma in adults. On both visual and dermoscopic examination, these signs are periungual pigmentation, variation of the degree of the pigmentation within the melanonychia, and color changes with aging.

B.M. Piraccini (✉) • A. Alessandrini • E. Dika • M. Starace
Department of Specialised Experimental and Diagnostic Medicine, Dermatology,
University of Bologna, Bologna, Italy
e-mail: biancamaria.piraccini@unibo.it

© Springer International Publishing Switzerland 2017
N. Di Chiacchio, A. Tosti (eds.), *Melanonychias*,
DOI 10.1007/978-3-319-44993-7_8

Unfortunately, no absolute criteria have been established to help definitively differentiate benign and malignant lesions in children on clinical and dermoscopic grounds. A "wait-and-see" approach to managing melanonychia in children is the most frequently suggested by nail experts, although this should include a prolonged follow-up using non-invasive techniques such as photography and dermoscopy. A correct clinical history and careful examination help the clinician to distinguish the different conditions and to decide on the correct management of melanonychia in children.

Epidemiology

Little has been published on the epidemiology of melanonychia in children (Baran 2012). It is generally rare and more common in pigmented races than in Caucasians. Melanonychia frequently appears as a longitudinal pigmented band within the nail plate, running from the proximal to the distal nail plate, involving a single digit. The fingernails are more frequently affected than the toenails, and among the fingernails, that on the first digit is most frequently affected. The mean age at onset is 3 years. The prevalence increases after puberty. No gender differences are reported among children.

Melanonychia in children is possibly due to melanocytic activation or melanocytic benign or malignant proliferation, as seen in adults. The most important causes of melanocytic activation are race, underlying syndromes, or drugs. Reactive nail pigmentation is extremely rare and several nails are usually involved. LM in children younger than 12 is not common in any race, especially in the fair-skinned population. No cases have been reported in the Chinese population younger than the age of 20 years (Leung et al. 2007), whereas 2.5% of black children younger than the age of 4 years have melanonychia (Leyden et al. 1972). In dark-skinned populations, such as African–Americans and people from the Caribbean, 77% of children have melanonychia caused by melanocytic activation, especially racial activation, but it is still rare to see under the age of 10 years. In these populations, racial melanonychia gradually appears with pigmented streaks in the nail after 10–12 years, whereas in the other dark-skinned races, it is possible to see the same pattern, but with an increased prevalence as a benign phenomenon with aging. Instead, in Caucasian and fair-skinned populations, the presence of pigmented streaks in children is caused by melanocytic proliferation. This type of melanonychia is a challenge both for the clinician and the pathologists to rule out melanoma in children, because melanonychia in a single digit in Caucasian children may represent an early subungual melanoma. The prevalence of this is remote and extremely rare, but cases have been reported.

Melanocytic proliferation is possible owing to benign melanocytic hyperplasia or nevus of the nail matrix. The first type was diagnosed in 30% of children with LM and the second type in 48% (Tosti et al. 1996; Goettmann-Bonvallott et al. 1999).

A clinical, histopathological, and outcome study of melanonychia in childhood was recently published. This study of 30 children showed that 20 cases were lentigo, five were subungual nevus, and the last five cases were melanocytic hyperplasia. All the cases were histologically confirmed (Cooper et al. 2015).

In the literature, only 12 cases of nail melanoma in children have been described.

History

Malignant and benign nail melanonychia are exceedingly rare in children. The most frequent form is nail matrix melanocytic nevus.

From a clinical point of view, it may be difficult to distinguish LM due to nevus from LM caused by other conditions, including nail melanoma. Management of melanonychia in children is not easy. The real problem for the clinicians is the atypical clinical and dermoscopic features that are considered possible indicators of nail unit melanoma in adults, which are frequently observed in benign melanocytic hyperplasia and nevi in children. The advice of the nail experts is to follow the patient periodically and decide after puberty whether or not to perform a tangential biopsy (Piraccini and Starace 2014).

Clinical Features

Melanonychia in children refers to black–brown–gray pigmentation of the nail due to the presence of melanin within the nail plate. It most frequently presents as a longitudinal band (LM) (Fig. 8.1a), but it may have a transversal aspect (transversal melanonychia) or involve the whole nail plate (total melanonychia) (Fig. 8.2). Melanonychia can involve one digit or several digits, both in the fingernails and in the toenails, and it appears at any age, from birth to adolescence. Normally in children, as in adults, nail matrix melanocytes are inactivated. Whatever the trigger factor that starts the production of melanin, it causes an activation or proliferation. The clinical aspect of melanonychia is different on the basis of the process involved.

- When multiple nails are involved in melanonychia, it is important to consider a normal racial variant, particularly in a dark-skinned population (Fig. 8.3), or that it represents one of the multiple signs of a syndrome. The syndromes that involve melanonychia in children are Peutz–Jeghers syndrome and Laugier–Hunziker syndrome. In the former, pigmented macules on the oral mucosa, lips, fingers, and toes, and melanonychia are associated with intestinal polyposis with a possible malignant degeneration. In Laugier–Hunziker syndrome, LM affects several nails and is associated with pigmented macules of the lips, mouth, esophageal mucosa, and genitalia. Other causes of melanocytic activation in children are trauma, irradiation, gold therapy, or treatment with cytotoxic agents. This type of activation usually affects the thumbs and index fingers. It is rare in children, but there are a few medications that have been reported to induce nail pigmentation. These include doxorubicin or hydroxyurea (M I and Khairkar 2003; Issaivanan et al. 2004). Rare cases are due to minocycline, zidovudine for ART therapy in

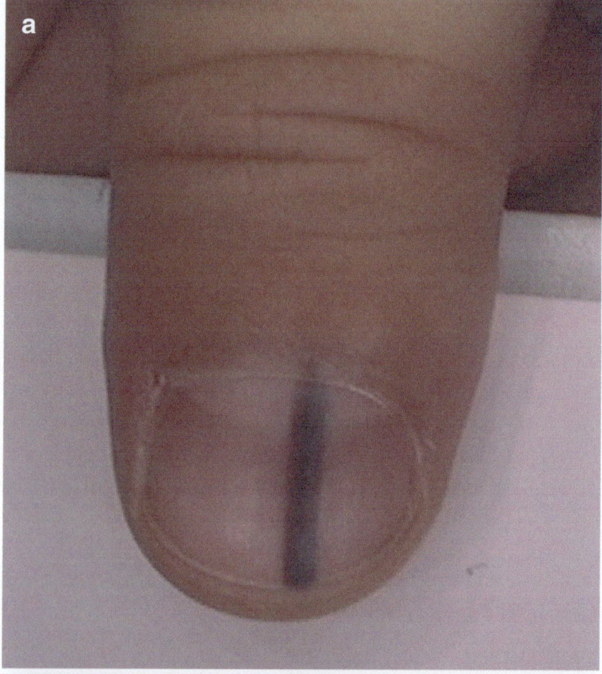

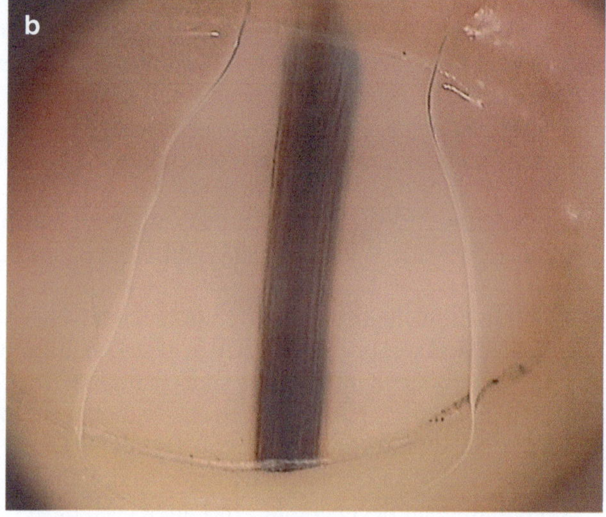

Fig. 8.1 Longitudinal melanonychia due to a nail matrix nevus in an 18-month-old child. (**a**) Clinical image revealing pseudo-Hutchinson's sign, which results from visualization of the nail plate pigmentation through the transparent cuticle. (**b**) Dermoscopy shows a brown background of the band, with lines irregular in width along their length

HIV patients, antimalarials, or cancer chemotherapeutics (Chen et al. 2007; Chawre et al. 2012). Melanonychia in children may also be a sign of arsenic intoxication, hemochromatosis, Addison's disease, or vitamin B12 deficiency (Baran and Kachijian 1989; Leung and Kao 2001). Dermoscopic patterns that suggest a melanocytic activation include a gray background of the band with thin, grayish, regular, and parallel lines (Fig. 8.4)

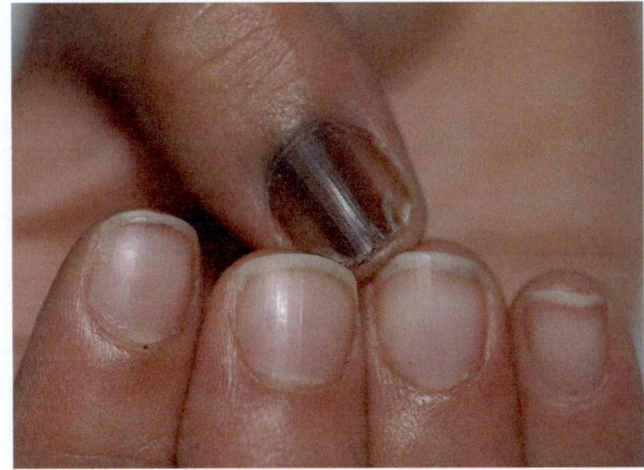

Fig. 8.2 Total melanonychia due to a nevus of the nail matrix in a 9-year-old girl. Clinical image shows a *brown* to *black* color and irregular longitudinal lines. The distal nail plate shows horizontal splitting

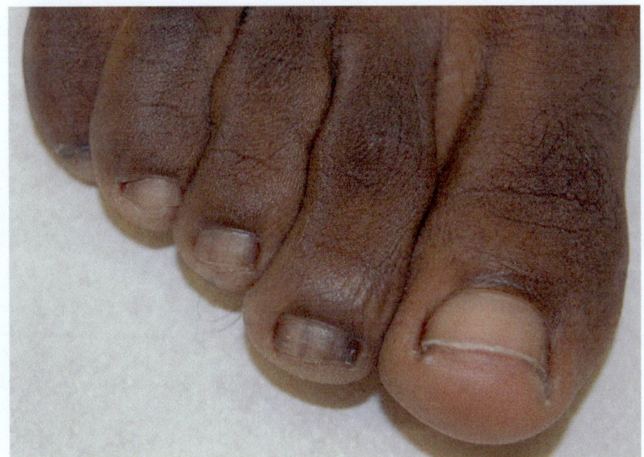

Fig. 8.3 Melanonychia of several toenails due to melanocyte activation in a dark-skinned adult

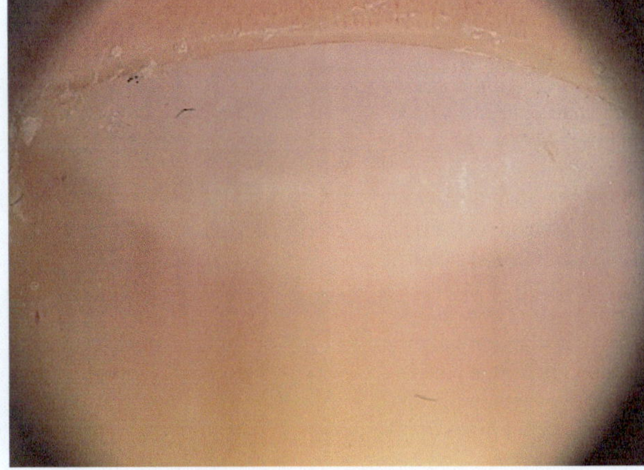

Fig. 8.4 Longitudinal melanonychia by melanocytic activation due to drugs. Dermoscopic image shows a *light brown* to *gray* background and thin regular lines

- When only one digit is involved in melanonychia, a proliferative process must be considered and a diagnostic dilemma of benign or malignant origin is posed. Usually, melanonychia due to proliferation appears with a longitudinal pigmented band. The aspect of the band may be very different: the color may be more or less pronounced and homogeneous, the borders may be well-defined or less sharp, and the width may range from a few millimeters to the entire nail plate. The corresponding nail plate may show some changes or be completely normal. Finally, a brown–black periungual pigmentation (Hutchinson's sign) may be present or absent (Fig. 8.5a). It is particularly important to examine all the aspects of melanonychia in children when a single digit is involved (Richert and André 2011). This recommendation is more important if the patient is a child, because the clinical and dermoscopic criteria that permit a clear differentiation in adults of benign to malignant lesions are not defined in pediatric patients. The clinical features of melanonychia in children are the same as in

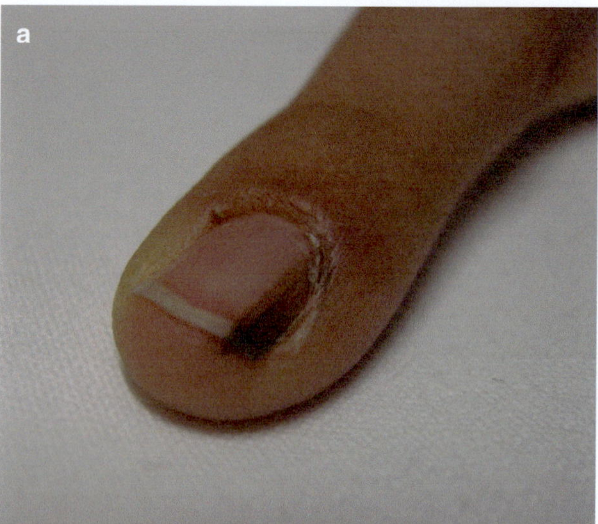

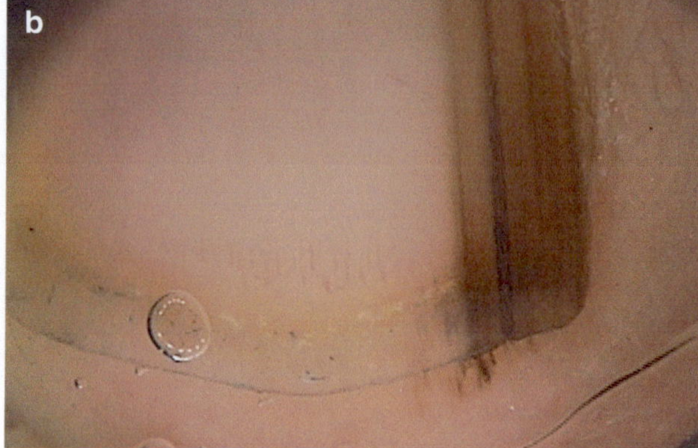

Fig. 8.5 Longitudinal melanonychia due to nevus of the nail matrix in an 11-year old boy. (**a**) Clinical image revealing irregular pigmentation of the nail plate associated with pigmentation of the hyponychium and proximal nail fold. (**b**) Dermoscopy shows Hutchinson's sign with parallel ridge pattern on the hyponychium and darker irregular lines on the nail plate

adults, but the most important difference is the extreme variability of the dimensions, degree of the pigmentation, and distribution of the pigment.

1. Nail matrix nevi are typically seen in childhood and may be congenital or acquired. Nail matrix nevi may be present at birth or they may develop at 2–4 years of age. Nail matrix nevi occur more frequently in fingernails than in toenails, most often in the thumb. The nail has one or more longitudinal, heavily pigmented bands. The size and the degree of pigmentation of the band of LM vary considerably among patients. The width of the band may vary in size from a few millimeters to the whole nail and the color may or may not be homogeneous and dark (Tosti et al. 2009). Over 50% of cases measure more than 3 mm (Goettmann-Bonvallott et al. 1999; Richert and André 2011). Dark bands are associated with pseudo-Hutchinson's sign, because the dark nail plate pigmentation is visible through the transparent nail fold (Fig. 8.1). The pigmentation may be homogeneously distributed or darker bands may appear over diffuse pale pigmentation. Some clinical features of nail matrix nevi in children can be alarming. The periungual pigmentation, Hutchinson's sign, is typical in congenital nevi and may involve both the nail proximal fold and the hyponychium (Fig. 8.5). It occurs in about a third of cases and is due to nests in the periungual epidermis and dermis. In children, it is not uncommon to notice a gradual enlargement of the band that may have a proximal part broader than the distal part (triangular). Darkening and spreading of the pigmentation is not unusual either. Thinning and fissuring of the pigmented nail plate may also occur. In children, it is quite common to observe a gradual fading of the band (Tosti et al. 1994). Fading of the pigmentation, called "regressing nevoid nail melanoma in childhood" is unique to children and not indicative of regression of the nevus, but may simply indicate a decrease in melanocytic activity from nevus cells (Kikuchi et al. 1993). A new dermoscopic sign that can indicate regression with fading of LM is the presence of dots, similar to that seen in skin lesions, distributed along melanocytic lines. In a recent Japanese study, 15 children were observed over a period of 2 years, and the authors noticed a gradual fading of LM in eight patients. These dots are black and have a regular size and shape from round to oval (less than 0.1 mm). The dots are distributed along the lines without regular distribution and sometimes they form a shallow pit at the periphery; at other times, it is possible to find them within the pigmented lines or interrupting the lines. In most young patients, the dots disappear over time. The authors explained the presence of dots as an accumulation of melanin derived from a cluster of nevus cells that migrate upward from the dermoepidermal junction. The fading of melanonychia occurs at the same time as the dots disappear. Thus, these dots are a sign of the regression of a nevus and not a warning sign of a melanoma (Murata and Kumano 2012). Dermoscopic patterns that suggest a nevus are the presence of a brown background and longitudinal brown to black regular and parallel lines with regular spacing and thickness, and, more importantly in children, black dots due to pigment accumulation in the nail plate (Fig. 8.6). Pathologically, most of the nevi in children are junctional nevi. Histological distinction between nail nevi and

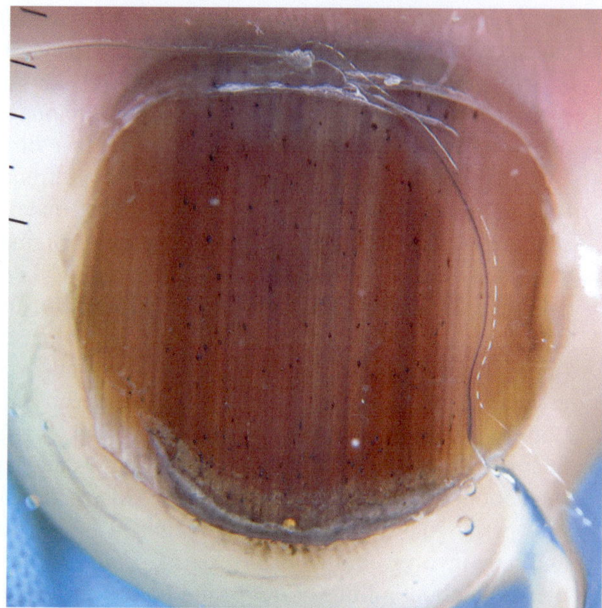

Fig. 8.6 Longitudinal melanonychia due to a nail matrix nevus in a 5-year-old child. Dermoscopy shows a brown background with regular lines and diffuse *dots* within the lines. Note the presence of pigmentation of the hyponychium

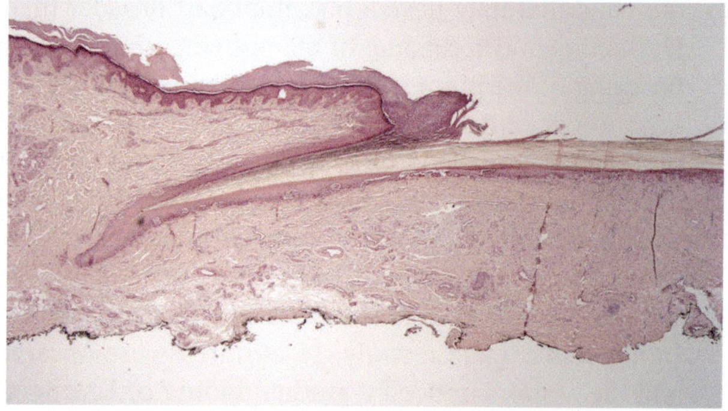

Fig. 8.7 Histopathology of a junctional nevus showing nests and melanocytes at the dermoepidermal junction

nail melanoma in children is not always easy. The most frequent situation is a nevus with nests at the dermoepidermal junction (Fig. 8.7). In this case, histological features are similar to those of acral nevi, with a lentiginous pattern of growth of melanocytes in early lesions (Di Chiacchio et al. 2013). To be sure of the benignity of the lesion, three characteristics suited to this region should be added. Nail matrix nevi are usually junctional, with regular nests and typical melanocytes; if there are zones of focal cytoplasmic dendrites, the distribution of the pigment may be uneven and the symmetrical aspect of the nevus may be seen only with great difficulty. Less frequently, it is possible to see a nevus without nests and it may be easily mistaken for the atypical aspect of melanocytes in the absence of nests that usually indicate a nevus. Major attention is advised to be given to the atypia of melanocytes where the atypical aspect is not atypical, but it is due to the enlarged form and vertical orientation with slightly pleomorphic cells separated from each other by a few basal keratinocytes. It is possible for all these aspects to be present in nail melanoma, but in differentiating them from "atypical melanocyte hyperplasia," the definition of the type of pleomorphic cells remains elusive (Perrin 2013).

2. Twelve cases of nail melanoma in children have been described in the literature. Eight of these reports are in Japanese children (Lyall 1967; Uchiyama and Minemura 1979), two are from South America, from Argentina and Brazil (Iorizzo et al. 2008), and the last two cases occurred in Caucasians (Tosti et al. 2012). Melanonychia is the presenting symptom that usually appears as a longitudinal band dark-brown in color with the presence of Hutchinson's sign (Antonovich et al. 2005). In general, only three of the Japanese cases were melanoma in situ of the nail apparatus: Kato et al. described a 2-year-old child (Kato et al. 1989), Kiryu et al. described a 3-year-old girl (Kiryu 1998), and Hori et al. a 3-year-old girl (Hori et al. 1988). The other cases described in Japanese children are melanonychia, which started to appear between the age of 1 month and 2 years. They changed after a follow-up period of 3–11 years into melanoma and lymph node metastases following a minor injury after the age of 20. In all these pigmented nails, there was a process of evolution or sometimes regression. Even if progression of melanoma is described, in all nail pigmentations in children, the histological examination reveals melanocytic nevi (Antonovich et al. 2005). The rate of progression of nail matrix nevi to melanoma is not known, but it is probably low. Thus, the main problem remains whether a benign lesion that appears in childhood can become a malignant lesion in adulthood. Dermoscopic patterns suggest that a melanoma might have a brown background with longitudinal, brown to black lines with irregular degrees of color pigmentation, spacing or varying thickness, and end abruptly or have a parallelism disruption. However, these features can also be seen in LM in children and the specificity at a young age is very low. The Japanese school in 2009 proposed an objective discrimination index (DI) for the differentiation of nail melanoma in situ from benign LM with the evaluation of dermatoscopic images (Koga et al. 2014). This study analyzed the variegation in a color image measured by the variety of the directions of pixel color vectors, but it was performed in adults with 100% sensitivity and 92% specificity. They recently proposed to apply the same DI of LM in 15 children and adolescents. According to their results the DI of LM exceeded the threshold value used in adults (Koga et al. 2016).

Diagnostic Clues

The correct approach to managing melanonychia in children does not exist, but the need to find it is very important, first of all, because of the anxiety of the parent. Parental anxiety around melanonychia is a consequence of the possible diagnosis of melanoma.

In a case of melanonychia in children, on the one hand, there is the remote risk of discovering a melanoma even if the overwhelming majority of pediatric cases are benign; on the other hand, there is the risk of sedation or anesthesia for an invasive procedure and possibly permanent nail dystrophy after surgery (Chu and Rubin 2014). It is important that this decision is taken by parents along with a nail expert dermatologist. Furthermore, there is the worry that a lesion that may be benign in childhood has the possible potential to evolve over time (Leclère et al. 2011).

The approach advised in case of melanonychia in children is to combine personal/family history together with clinical and dermoscopic features. These three components provide an insight into the differential diagnosis of melanonychia in addition to the decision to perform a biopsy. Dermoscopy is a non-invasive technique that enhances the clinical evaluation of LM and has been demonstrated to be helpful in improving the clinical decision-making regarding whether or not to perform a biopsy (Adigun and Scher 2012; Baran 1993). The role of dermoscopy in the follow-up of these lesions is still not established; the best way to manage these patients is to repeat a regular and accurate follow-up that includes global photography and video dermoscopy with storage of images on a computer. According to the literature, the dermatologist should advise immediate excision of pigmented lesions with alarming clinical features such as a band that enlarges to involve the whole nail plate and/or darkens, and/or bands with irregular borders and spacing, and/or a thick pattern of lines and areas of parallelism disruption. The decision to perform a biopsy in a younger child with melanonychia is taken when the parents are very anxious. In general, it is recommended to excise all bands as a preventative measure after puberty. Tangential excision is the best option when surgery is chosen (Di Chiacchio et al. 2013).

Summary for the Clinician

Clinical features of melanonychia in children are variable according to the etiology. A thorough history, dermoscopy of the nail plate, and strict follow-up may aid in the diagnosis and management.

In children, signs that are frightening when present in adults are not considered worrisome. These signs can be present in benign lesions, especially nevi, but they cannot be overlooked. The current clinical and dermoscopic criteria for melanonychia in the adult population simply do not translate to the pediatric population.

Melanonychia in children requires a conservative approach, but a long-term follow-up is mandatory for the early detection of possible malignant changes. Evaluation of melanonychia in children is recommended every 6 months. It is important that these patients are followed by a dermatologist with nail expertise and advised to return for regular evaluation if the lesion shows any quick changes during this time. Any case of melanonychia in children with clinical and/or dermoscopic changes developed over a short period during follow-up, requires biopsy for histopathological examination.

References

Adigun CG, Scher RK. Longitudinal melanonychia: when to biopsy and is dermoscopy helpful? Dermatol Ther. 2012;25:491–7.

Antonovich DD, Grin C, Grant-Kels JM. Childhood subungual melanoma in situ in diffuse nail melanosis beginning as expanding longitudinal melanonychia. Pediatr Dermatol. 2005;22:210–2.

Baran R. Longitudinal melanonychia. Dermatology. 1993;186:83.

Baran R, de Berker DAR, Holzberg M, Thomas L. Baran and Dawber's diseases of the nails and their management. 4th ed. New York: Wiley-Blackwell; 2012.

Baran B, Kachijian P. Longitudinal melanonychia (melanonychia striata): diagnosis and management. J Am Acad Dermatol. 1989;21:1165–75.

Chawre S, Pore SM, Nandeshwar MB, Masood NM. Zidovudine-induced nail pigmentation in a 12-year-old boy. Indian J Pharm. 2012;44:801–2.

Chen W, Yu YS, Liu YH, Sheen JM, Hsiao CC. Nail changes associated with chemotherapy in children. J Eur Acad Dermatol Venereol. 2007;21:186–90.

Chu DH, Rubin AI. Diagnosis and management of nail disorders in children. Pediatr Clin. 2014;61:293–308.

Cooper C, Arva NC, Lee C, Yélamos O, Obregon R, Sholl LM, Wagner A, Shen L, Guitart JP. A clinical, histopathologic, and outcome study of melanonychia striata in childhood. J Am Acad Dermatol. 2015;72(5):773–9.

Di Chiacchio N, Ruben BS, Loureiro WR. Longitudinal melanonychias. Clin Dermatol. 2013;31:594–601.

Goettmann-Bonvallott S, André J, Belaich S. Longitudinal melanonychia in children: a clinical and histopathologic study of 40 cases. J Am Acad Dermatol. 1999;41:17–22.

Hori Y, Yamada A, Tanizaki T. Pigmented small tumors. Jpn J Pediatr Dermatol. 1988;7:117–20.

Iorizzo M, Tosti A, Di Chiacchio N, et al. Nail melanoma in children: differential diagnosis and management. Dermatol Surg. 2008;34:974–8.

Issaivanan M, Mitu PS, Manisha C, Praveen K. Cutaneous manifestations of hydroxyurea therapy in childhood: case report and review. Pediatr Dermatol. 2004;21:124–7.

Kato T, Usuba Y, Takematsu H, et al. A rapidly growing pigmented nail streak resulting in diffuse melanosis of the nail. A possible sign of subungual melanoma in situ. Cancer. 1989;64:2191–8.

Kikuchi I, Inoue S, Sakaguchi E, et al. Regressing nevoid nail melanosis in childhood. Dermatology. 1993;186:88–93.

Kiryu H. Malignant melanoma in situ arising in the nail unit of a child. J Dermatol. 1998;25:41–4.

Koga H, Yoshikawa S, Shinohara T, Sekiguchi A, Fujii J, Saida T, Sota T. An automated evaluation system of dermoscopic images of longitudinal melanonychia: proposition of a discrimination index for detecting early nail apparatus melanoma. J Dermatol. 2014;41:867–71.

Koga H, Yoshikawa S, Shinohara T, Le Gal FA, Cortés B, Saida T, Sota T. Long-term follow–up of longitudinal melanonychia in children and adolescent using an objective discrimination index. Acta Derm Venereol. 2016;96:716.

Leclère FM, Mordon S, Leroy M, Lefebvre C, Schoofs M. Presentation, microsurgical therapy, and clinical outcomes in three patients of expanding melanonychia of the nail unit in children. Arch Orthop Trauma Surg. 2011;131:1453–7.

Leung AK, Kao CP. An atlas of nail disorders. Consultant. 2001;41:58–64.

Leung AK, Robson WL, Liu EK, Kao CP, Fong JH, Leong AG, Cheung BC, Wong AH, Chen SY. Melanonychia striata in Chinese children and adults. Int J Dermatol. 2007;46:920–2.

Leyden JJ, Spott DA, Goldschmidt H. Diffuse and banded melanin pigmentation in nails. Arch Dermatol. 1972;105:548–50.

Lyall D. Malignant melanoma in infancy. J Am Med Assoc. 1967;202:93.

M I, Khairkar PH. Doxorubicin induced melanonychia. Indian Pediatr. 2003;40:1094–5.

Murata Y, Kumano K. Dots and lines: a dermoscopic sign of regression of longitudinal melanonychia in children. Cutis. 2012;90:293–6.

Perrin C. Tumors of the nail unit. A review. I. Acquired localized longitudinal melanonychia and erythronychia. Am J Dermatopathol. 2013;6:621–36.

Piraccini BM, Starace M. Nail disorders in infants and children. Dermatology. 2014;26:1–6.

Richert B, André J. Nail disorders in children: diagnosis and management. Am J Acad Dermatol. 2011;12:101–12.

Tosti A, Baran R, Morelli R, et al. Progressive fading of a longitudinal melanonychia due to a nail matrix melanocytic naevus in a child. Arch Dermatol. 1994;130:1076–7.

Tosti A, Baran R, Piraccini BM, et al. Nail matrix nevi: a clinical and histopathologic study of 22 patients. J Am Acad Dermatol. 1996;34:765–71.

Tosti A, Piraccini BM, Cadore de Farias D. Dealing with melanonychia. Semin Cutan Med Surg. 2009;28:49–54.

Tosti A, Piraccini BM, Cagalli A, et al. In situ melanoma of the nail unit in children: report pf two cases in fair-skinned Caucasian children. Pediatr Dermatol. 2012;29:79–83.

Uchiyama M, Minemura K. Two cases of malignant melanoma in young persons. Nippon Hifuka Gakkai Zasshi. 1979;89:668.

Non-melanocytic Melanonychia

Anna Q. Hare, Emily Bolton, and Phoebe Rich

> **Key Features**
> Nonmelanocytic causes of melanonychia include exogenous and endogenous factors.
>
> Monodactylous versus polydactylous pathology is helpful in narrowing the differential diagnosis.
>
> The presence of key findings on physical examination may point to a diagnosis.
>
> Non-invasive diagnostic procedures can preclude the need for biopsy.
>
> Caution is always warranted as multiple pathological conditions can coexist in the nail, and it is recommended to follow any nail pigmentation over time.

Introduction

Melanonychia is brown, black, or gray pigmentation of the nail of any cause. Most cases of melanonychia are the result of increased production of melanin by nail matrix melanocytes because of either melanocyte activation or melanocyte proliferation. In some cases, melanonychia is caused by substances other than melanin, such as blood, fungi, or pyocyanin produced from *Pseudomonas aeruginosa*. Often, these other

A.Q. Hare, MD
Department of Dermatology, Oregon Health and Science University, CHH16D, 3303 SW Bond Avenue, Portland, OR 97239, USA

E. Bolton, MS
Creighton University School of Medicine, 2500 California Plaza, Omaha, NE 68178, USA

P. Rich, MD (✉)
Department of Dermatology, Oregon Health and Science University, 2565 NW Lovejoy St., Portland, Oregon
e-mail: phoeberich@aol.com

© Springer International Publishing Switzerland 2017
N. Di Chiacchio, A. Tosti (eds.), *Melanonychias*,
DOI 10.1007/978-3-319-44993-7_9

pigments mimic the clinical features of nail melanoma; therefore, careful diagnosis and workup are important. If the cause of melanonychia is not clinically clear, additional measures must be taken to determine whether the pigmentation is derived from matrix melanocytes or from other sources. Knowledge of these diverse etiologies of melanonychia is important to thoroughly work up melanonychia in a patient. Discussions in this chapter focus mainly on nail pigmentation from causes not directly related to matrix melanocyte melanin production, although there is some overlap.

It is convenient to discuss melanonychia in terms of causes that are exogenous or endogenous to the nail. Exogenous causes include local infection, trauma, and staining; endogenous processes include medications, inflammation, and hormones.

Epidemiology

Melanonychia not caused by melanoma or melanocyte activation is very common. Although those with a darker complexion have a higher propensity toward melanocyte activation, exogenous causes such as trauma, infection with fungus or bacteria, or exogenous staining have no boundaries within the population. However, knowing the medical background, occupation, and hobbies of the patient may help to point toward certain etiologies. Patients with diabetes or HIV may be at a higher risk for fungal or bacterial infection, or may be taking medications known to cause melanonychia. Those whose occupations involve heavy metals or who frequently use staining products such as tobacco or hair dyes are obviously at a higher risk of nail pigmentation from those products.

Clinical Features

Organisms

The most common cause of exogenous nail pigmentation is fungal melanonychia. Dermatophytes are the most common organism responsible for onychomycosis

Table 9.1 Some common organisms causing fungal melanonychia

Dermatophyte molds
Trichophyton rubrum
Trichophyton soudanense
Yeasts
Candida albicans
Candida tropicalis
Candida parapsilosis
Nondermatophyte molds
Fusarium oxysporum
Chaetomium spp.
Scytalidium
Aspergillus niger
Cladosporium
Exophiala

(approximately 75% of all cases; yet, the causative organism can be yeast, dermatophytes, or nondermatophytic molds (Table 9.1) (Baran et al. 2012; Tosti 2015). In melanonychia caused by fungal infection, the organism itself is generally the source of the pigment. Many dermatophytes produce a soluble, nongranular melanin, either in their cell walls or excreted, that can stain the nail plate (Haneke and Baran 2001). It is hypothesized that there is an evolutionary advantage to melanin production among fungi, which may confer some resistance to some topical antifungal therapy (Baran et al. 2012). Dematiaceous fungi, which produce pigment, are increasingly common culprits in onychomycosis and are more resistant to treatment than typical dermatophytes. *Trichophyton rubrum*, a dermatophyte, and the dematiaceous non-dermatophyte mold *Scytalidium dimidiatum* are the most common agents of fungal melanonychia (Tosti 2015). One helpful finding in melanonychia due to fungal infection is that the melanonychia typically spares the matrix, whereas a neoplasm producing melanin commonly originates in the matrix. Occasionally, fungal stimulation of matrix melanocytes may be seen, causing longitudinal melanonychia that can make differentiation difficult. Other clues to dermatophytes being a cause of melanonychia include surrounding nail yellow dyschromia or subungual debris noted in multiple nails (Figs. 9.1, 9.2, 9.3, 9.4, and 9.5). When a fungal cause is suspected, a positive potassium hydroxide (KOH) test on a nail clipping is the first and easiest step in diagnosis, followed by culture, nail clipping for histology, and periodic acid-Schiff (PAS) or in some cases polymerase chain reaction (PCR) (Gupta and Simpson 2013; Stephen et al. 2015; Finch et al. 2012).

Several Gram-negative bacteria such as *Pseudomonas* and *Proteus* can cause melanonychia as well, which can be dark and sinister appearing in some nails (Haneke and Baran 2001). This pigmentation typically occurs at the lateral nail fold. *Pseudomonas*, the most common of these, affects onycholytic nails and deposits a green black pigment called pyocyanin. Treatment in this case consists of topical anti-pseudomonal medications, including eye drops and drying topical medications,

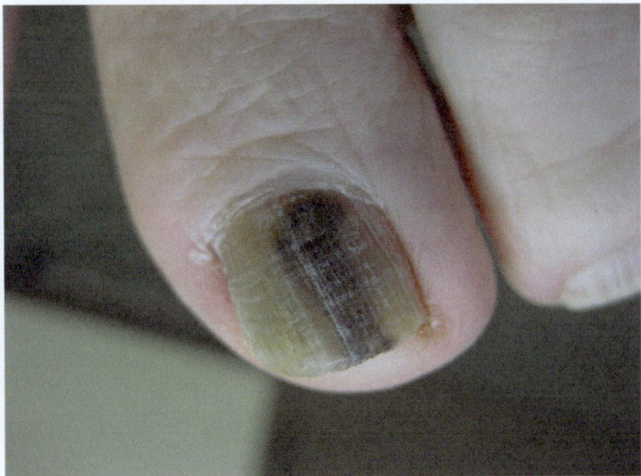

Fig. 9.1 Fungal melanonychia

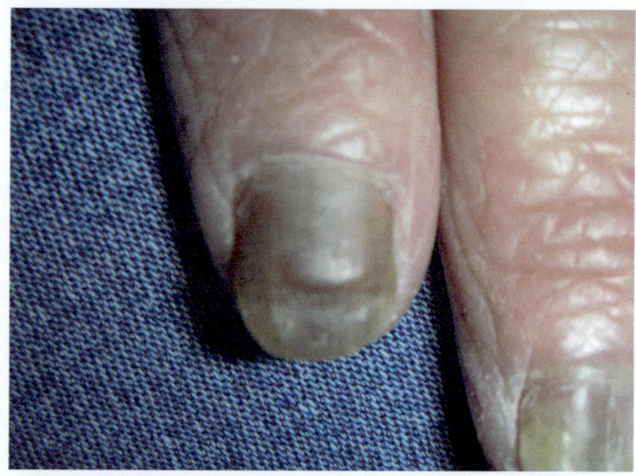

Fig. 9.2 Fungal melanonychia

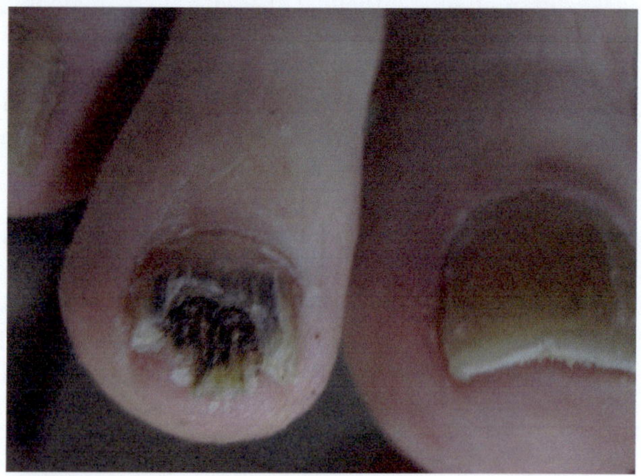

Fig. 9.3 Fungal melanonychia with the overlying nail plate removed

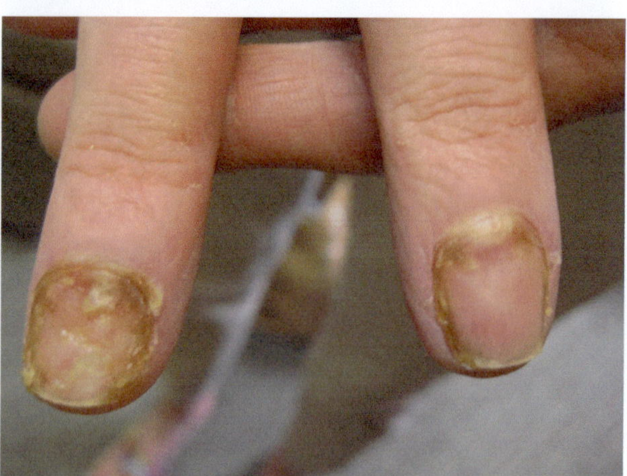

Fig. 9.4 Nondermatophyte mold as a cause of pigmentation

Fig. 9.5 Candida and paronychia

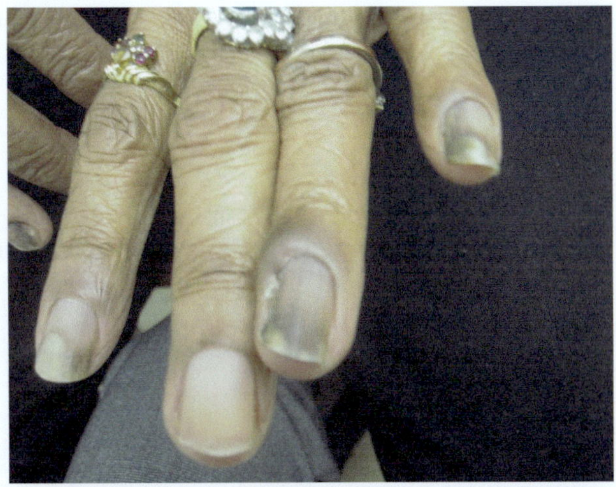

Fig. 9.6 Fungal melanonychia with onycholysis and *Pseudomonas*

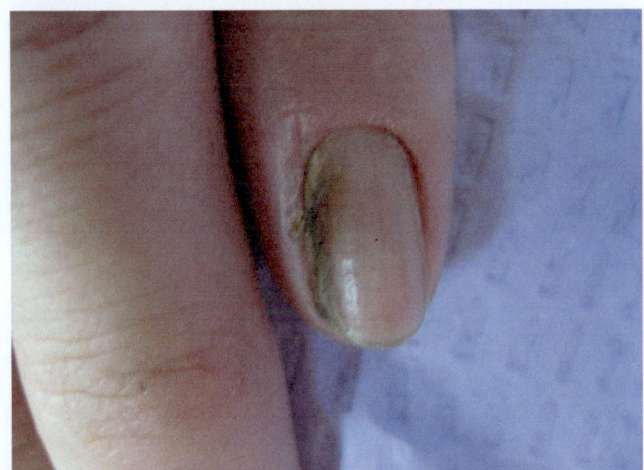

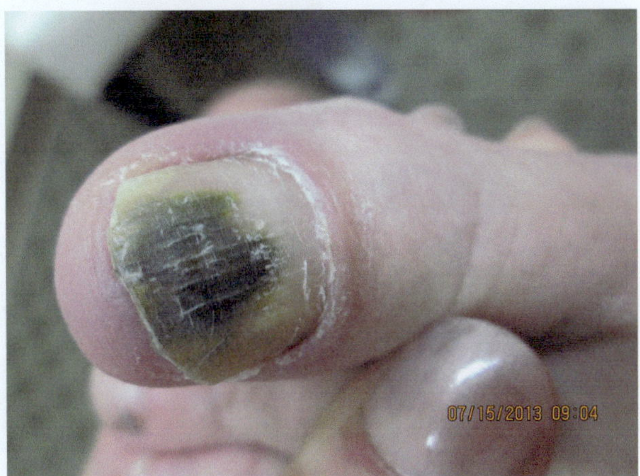

Fig. 9.7 Melanonychia due to *Pseudomonas* in an onycholytic nail

and treating any underlying onychomycosis and onycholysis of any cause is helpful (Figs. 9.6 and 9.7).

Trauma

Trauma can result in a dark nail, causing alarm among physicians and patients who worry that the black color is due to melanoma (Figs. 9.8 and 9.9). Trauma causes dark

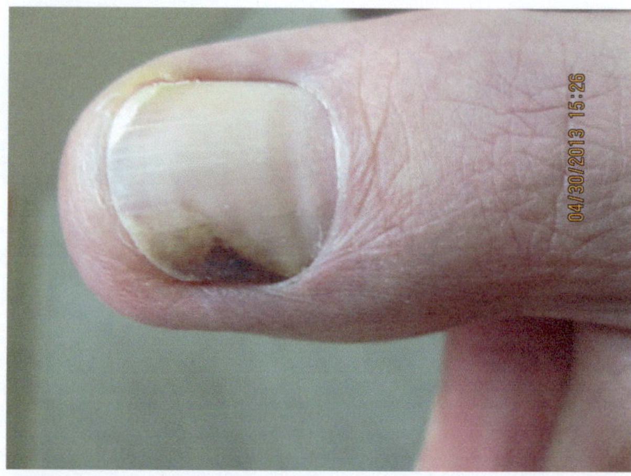

Fig. 9.8 Subungual hemorrhage: notice the sharp demarcation

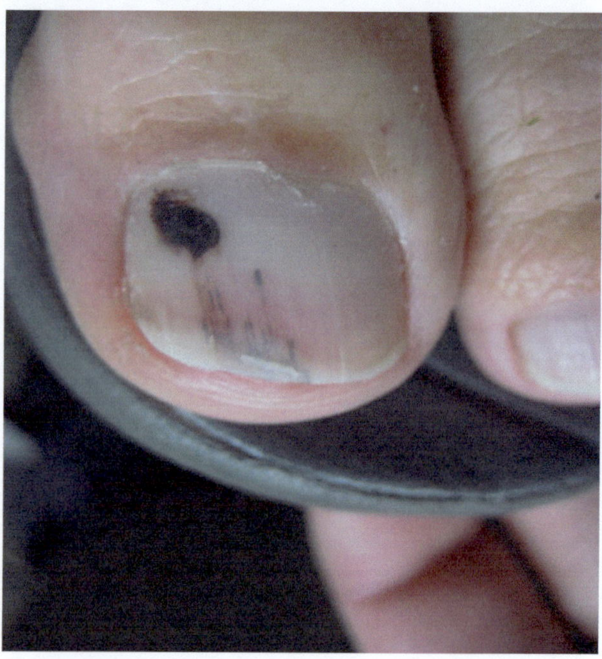

Fig. 9.9 Hemorrhage under the nail

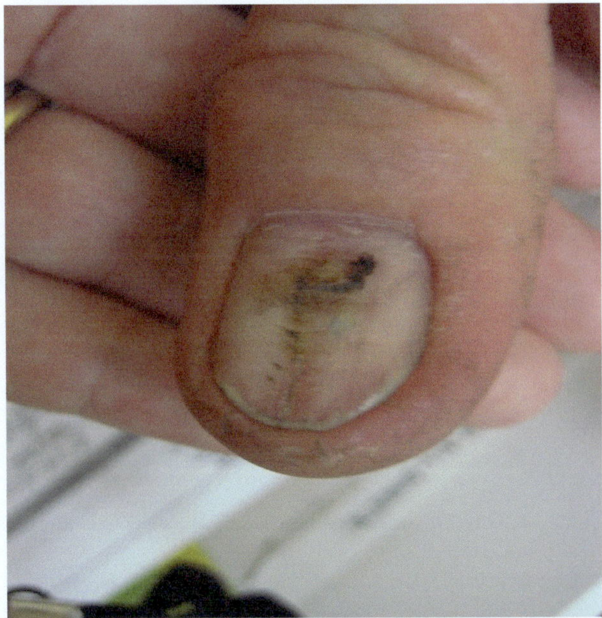

Fig. 9.10 Hemorrhage and habit tic dystrophy (chronic trauma)

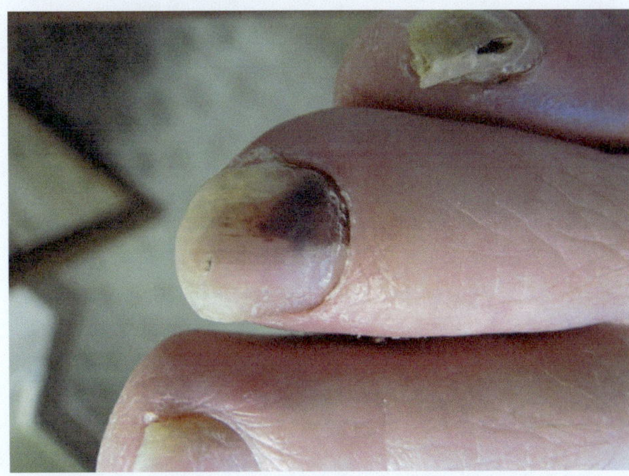

Fig. 9.11 Hemorrhage, notice that where the blood has washed away, the nail becomes onycholytic

nails in two ways: (1) via subungual blood or (2) via melanocyte activation. In the case of subungual blood, it is incumbent on the clinician to prove that the pigment is blood. The cause of subungual blood includes both acute trauma in addition to chronic, minor, repetitive trauma, which the patient may not recall (Fig. 9.10). If the trauma occurs in the proximal matrix, the blood may be incorporated into the nail plate in the top layers. If blood occurs in distal matrix or nail bed, the blood may leave a space as it dries and results in nail plate lifting as the nail grows out. This can create onycholysis as the blood is eventually washed away (Fig. 9.11). Clipping the overlying nail and examining it via microscopy can often give the diagnosis (Stephen et al. 2015)

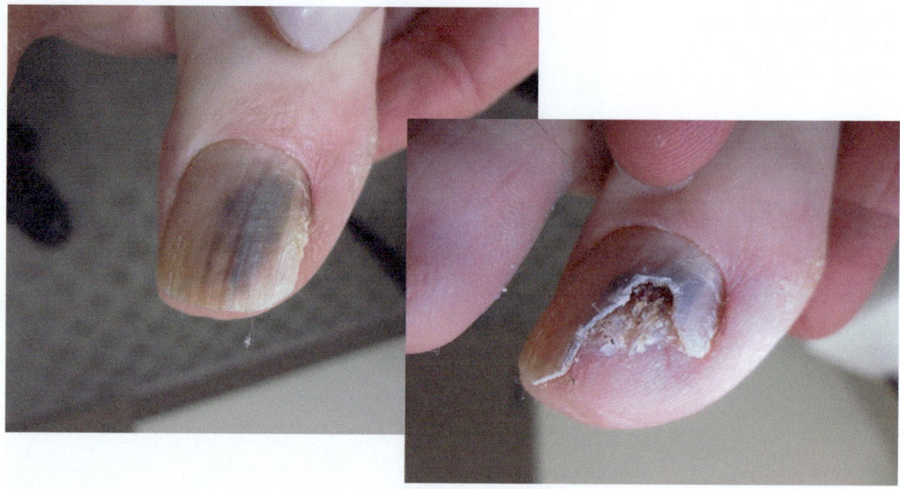

Fig. 9.12 Onycholytic nail painlessly clipped away to confirm the presence of hemorrhage

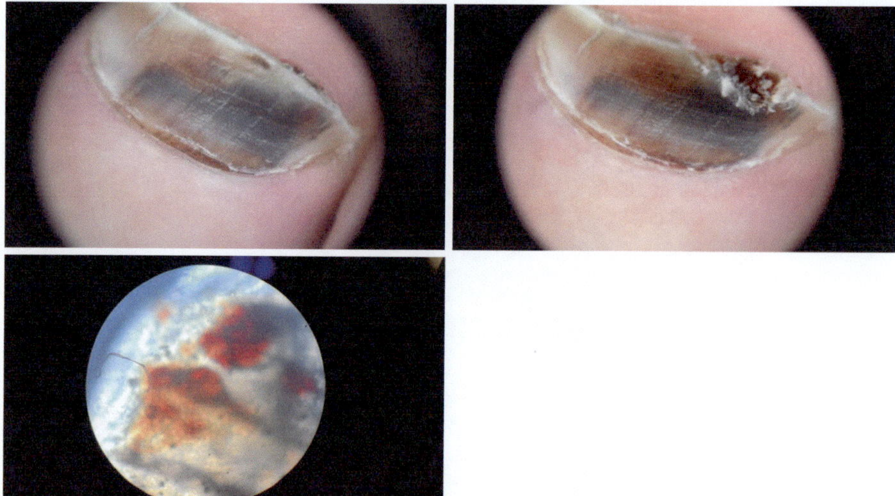

Fig. 9.13 Nail clipping revealing subungual blood

(Fig. 9.12). Dermoscopy of subungual blood is characterized by red–blue–black globules, longitudinal short streaks, and well-circumscribed blotches (Figs. 9.13 and 9.14). The pigmentation moves distally with nail growth and is replaced by normal colored nail at the proximal nail fold. This is in contrast to the dermatoscopic features of longitudinal melanonychia of melanoma, where longitudinal pigmentation that extends to the free edge of the nail is composed of multiple, irregular, brown–black lines within the broader area of pigmentation (Mun et al. 2013).

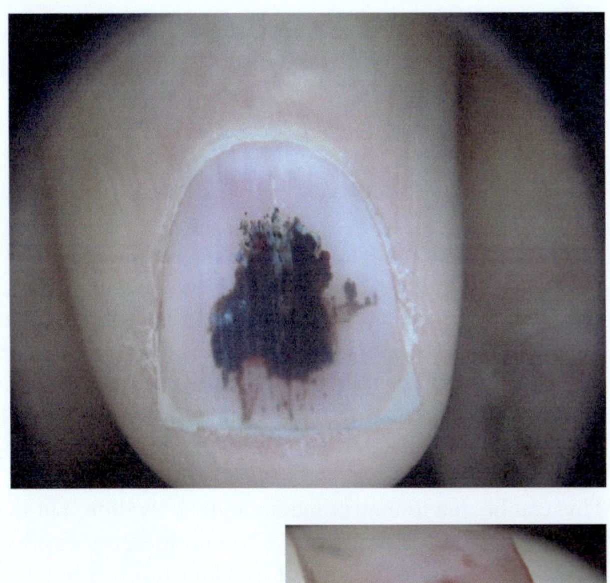

Fig. 9.14 Dermoscopy of subungual hemorrhage illustrating globules and streaks

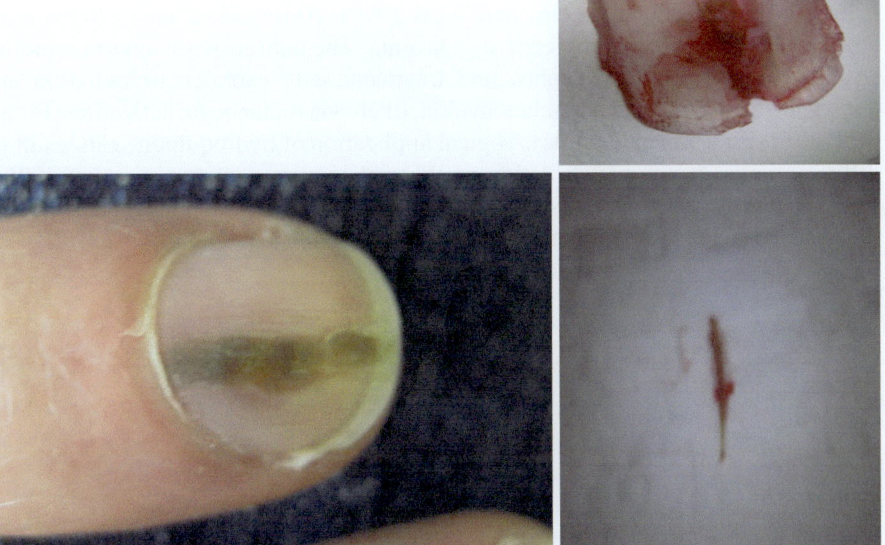

Fig. 9.15 Foreign body causing melanonychia: cactus spine

Trauma may also result in splinter hemorrhages, which are longitudinal collections of blood in the nail that appear black. These are rarely confused with melanoma or nevus because they do not span the length of the nail plate. Caution must be exercised, as blood does not exclude the presence of a tumor, as these can coexist (Fig. 9.15). Trauma may also result in the activation of matrix melanocytes, causing longitudinal melanonychia. This may occur with chronic nail tip trauma, friction, or picking.

Distinct from trauma is the presence of a foreign body under the nail plate, which can itself appear dark or may result in blood or infection under the nail plate that appears dark (Fig. 9.16).

Staining

A variety of external stains can cause melanonychia. Typically, multiple nails are involved. Silver nitrate, self-tanning creams, tar, iodine, and various other products can stain the surface of the nail and result in pigmentation (Baran et al. 2012). Although patient history and the involvement of multiple nails are keys to this diagnosis, one clue indicating an exogenous cause of pigmentation is that the proximal margin of the pigment remains in an arc shape parallel to the proximal nail fold as the nail plate grows (Baran et al. 2012) (Figs. 9.17, 9.18, and 9.19).

Some exogenous substances, when ingested, cause pigmentation in the nail. This can be due to matrix melanocyte activation, but may also be a direct effect of deposition into the nail plate. Chronic mercury exposure and other heavy metals can result in multiple bands of melanonychia. Some medications fall into this category, such as clofazimine, which deposits in the nail plate causing pigmentation (Piraccini et al. 2006; Piraccini and Tosti 1999). Antimalarial medications may also cause melanonychia via ferric dyschromia. The antiretroviral azidothymidine (AZT), chemotherapeutic agents, and treatment with psoralen or radiation are known to cause longitudinal melanonychia, likely via melanocyte activation (Baran et al. 2012; Piraccini et al. 2006). Topical application of hydroquinone can result in diffuse orange–brown pigmentation of the nails exposed (Piraccini et al. 2006). Anticoagulants can result in subungual hemorrhage and splinter hemorrhages in the absence of recalled trauma.

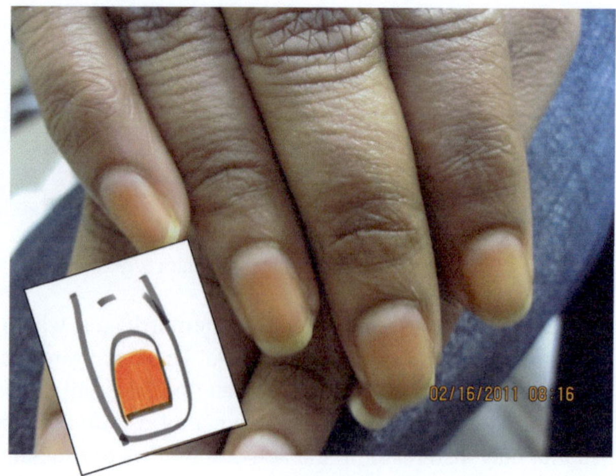

Fig. 9.16 Exogenous brown pigmentation. Notice that the proximal margin is parallel to the nail fold

Fig. 9.17 Staining from minocycline

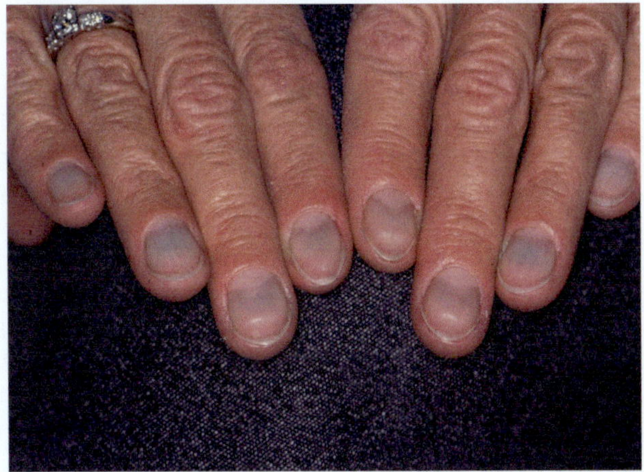

Fig. 9.18 Longitudinal melanonychia from hydroxyurea

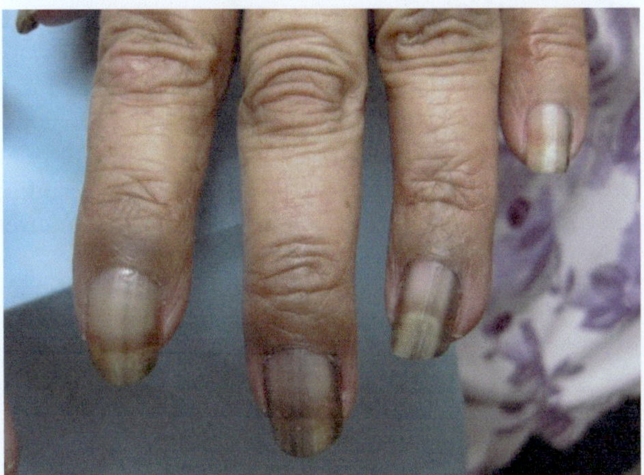

Fig. 9.19 Myxoid cyst with hemorrhage

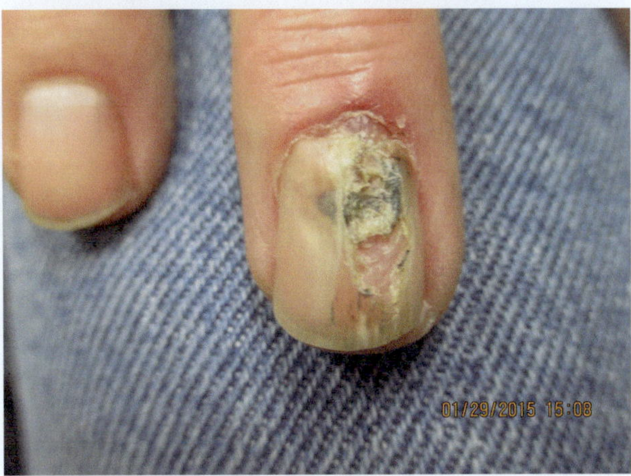

Neoplasms

Several nonmelanocytic nail tumors can present as longitudinal melanonychia and simulate melanoma. Pigmented Bowen's disease, onychomatricoma, mucous cyst, subungual fibrous histiocytoma, subungual linear keratotic melanonychia, and verruca vulgaris have been documented to cause longitudinal melanonychia (Baran et al. 2012; Stetsenko et al. 2008; Wynes et al. 2015; Baran and Simon 1988). Onychopapilloma can appear as a red band (due to thinning of the nail plate) or a dark band (due to blood in the channel beneath the nail plate) and may have splinter hemorrhages. Onychopapilloma often has a verrucous subungual papule visible at the free edge of the nail plate, as a key to diagnosis (Tosti et al. 2015). Occasionally, the streak of blood appears alarming to the physician, in which case the nail can be removed and the diagnosis confirmed (Figs. 9.15, 9.16, and 9.20).

Diagnostic Clues

Subungual melanoma is the most concerning and most feared cause of melanonychia. However, there are many more common causes of melanonychia. Using clinical signs to identify likely pathology and to preclude the need for a biopsy is an important skill. The following simple algorithm is one model for assessing the aforementioned signs of nonmelanocytic causes of melanonychia before biopsy.

Summary for the Clinician
1. Longitudinal pigmented bands in the nail may be caused by melanocytic and nonmelanocytic processes.
2. The most common and most important causes of nonmelanocytic melanonychia are subungual hemorrhage and fungal melanonychia.
3. Distinguishing subungual hemorrhage from nail melanoma by clinical, historical, and dermatoscopic features is very useful.
4. Recognizing the clinical and diagnostic features of nonmelanocytic melanonychia may help the clinician to arrive at the correct cause of aberrant pigment in the nail and possibly avoid unnecessary nail biopsy.

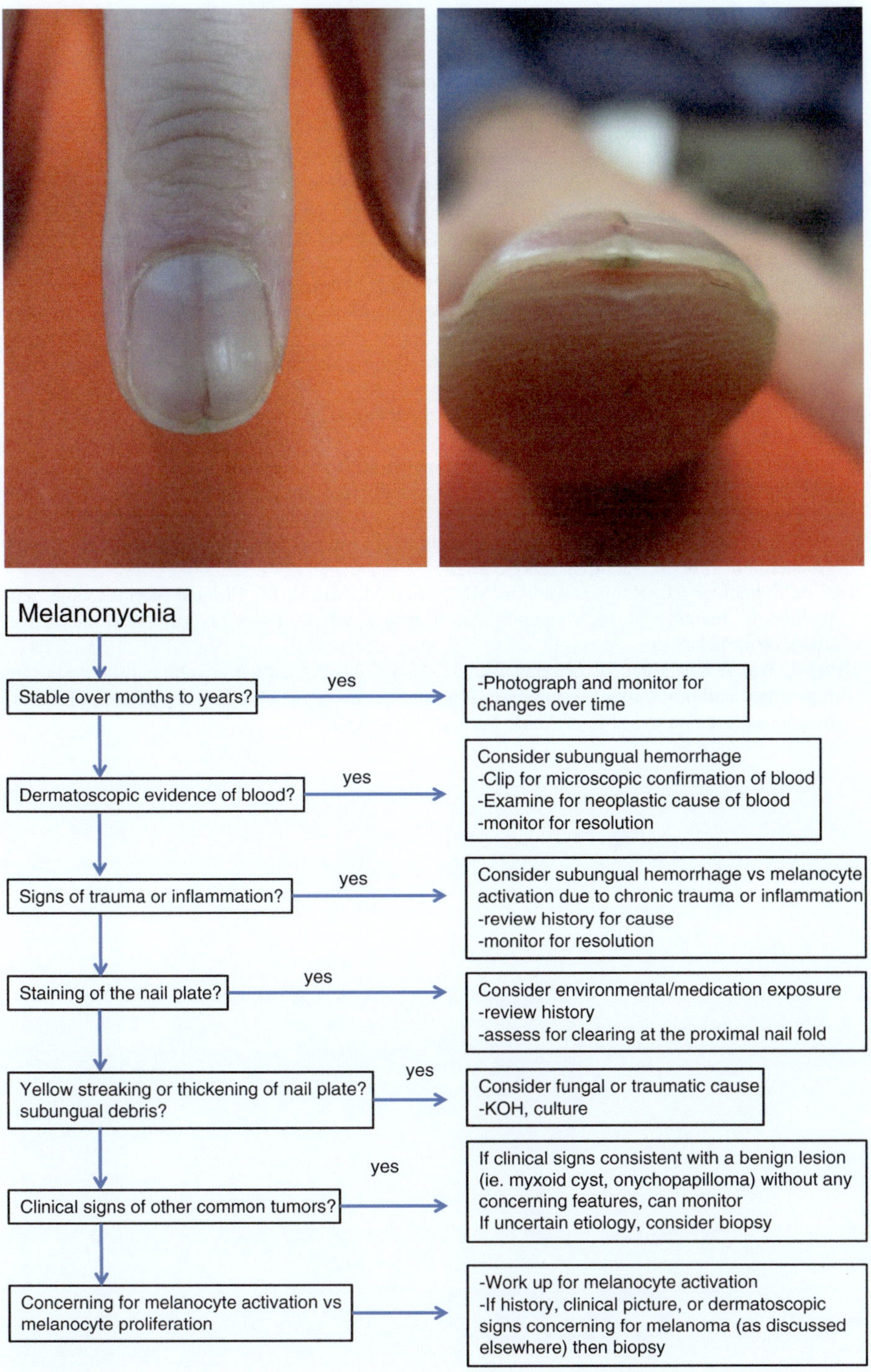

Fig. 9.20 Onychopapilloma with hemorrhage and with characteristic distal subungual hyperkeratotic papule

References

Baran R, Simon C. Longitudinal melanonychia: a symptom of Bowen's disease. J Am Acad Dermatol. 1988;18(6):1359–60.

Baran R, de Berker D, Holzberg M, Thomas L, editors. Baran and Dawber's diseases of the nails and their management. 4th ed. New York: Wiley-Blackwell; 2012.

Finch J, Arenas R, Baran R. Fungal melanonychia. J Am Acad Dermatol. 2012;66(5):830–41.

Gupta AK, Simpson FC. Diagnosing onychomycosis. Clin Dermatol. 2013;31(5):540–3.

Haneke E, Baran R. Longitudinal melanonychia. Dermatol Surg 2001;27(6):580–584.

Mun JH, Kim GW, Jwa SW, et al. Dermoscopy of subungual haemorrhage: its usefulness in differential diagnosis from nail-unit melanoma. British J Dermatol. 2013;168(6):1224–9.

Piraccini BM, Tosti A. Drug-induced nail disorders: incidence, management and prognosis. Drug Saf. 1999;21(3):187–201.

Piraccini BM, Iorizzo M, Starace M, Tosti A. Drug-induced nail diseases. Dermatol Clin. 2006;24(3):387–91.

Stephen S, Tosti A, Rubin AI. Diagnostic applications of nail clippings. Dermatol Clin. 2015;33(2):289–301.

Stetsenko GY, McFarlane RJ, Chien AJ, et al. Subungual Bowen disease in a patient with epidermodysplasia verruciformis presenting clinically as longitudinal melanonychia. Am J Dermatopathol. 2008;30(6):582–5.

Tosti A. Nail disorders: practical tips for diagnosis and treatment, an issue of dermatologic clinics. Amsterdam: Elsevier Health Sciences; 2015.

Tosti A, Schneider SL, Ramirez-Quizon MN, Zaiac M, Miteva M. Clinical, dermoscopic, and pathologic features of onychopapilloma: a review of 47 cases. J Am Acad Dermatol. 2016;74(3):521–526.

Wynes J, Wanat KA, Huen A, Mlodzienski AJ, Rubin AI. Pigmented onychomatricoma: a rare pigmented nail unit tumor presenting as longitudinal melanonychia that has potential for misdiagnosis as melanoma. J Foot Ankle Surg. 2015;54(4):723–5.

Histological Analysis of the Nail Plate in the Diagnosis of Melanonychia and Other Nail Pigmentation

Beth S. Ruben

> **Key Features**
> - Melanocytic activation is a common cause of pigmentation of the nail plate and consists of melanin production without a proliferation of melanocytes.
> - Melanocytic proliferations (lentigo, nevi, and melanoma) often produce a solitary longitudinal pigmented band, while melanocytic activation can produce a single or multiple bands.
> - Other causes of nail plate pigmentation: pigmented squamous cell carcinoma, pigmented onychomatricoma, onychocytic matricoma, pigmented onychomycosis, and nail plate hemorrhage.
> - Nail clipping can serve as a less invasive screening procedure for identifying the cause of nail plate discoloration.
> - Fontana–Masson staining is useful in identifying melanin.
> - A modified benzidine stain can be used to identify hemoglobin.

Introduction

Pigmentation of the nail plate is often due to melanin (melanonychia) and often arises from a melanocytic lesion producing melanin in the nail matrix. Such lesions are discussed in more detail elsewhere in this book. Melanocytic activation is a common cause of pigmentation and consists of melanin production without a proliferation of melanocytes. It may occur in a reactive manner owing to many disruptions of the nail unit, or it may be a primary condition creating a pigmented band or bands. Melanocytic proliferations such as lentigo (melanocytic hyperplasia), nevi, and melanoma often

B.S. Ruben, MD
Department of Dermatology, University of California, San Francisco, CA, USA

Dermatopathology Service, Palo Alto Medical Foundation, Palo Alto, CA, USA
e-mail: RubenBS@sutterhealth.org

© Springer International Publishing Switzerland 2017
N. Di Chiacchio, A. Tosti (eds.), *Melanonychias*,
DOI 10.1007/978-3-319-44993-7_10

produce a solitary longitudinal pigmented band (Ruben 2015). There are also other neoplastic causes of melanin pigmentation in the nail plate, such as pigmented squamous cell carcinoma (Baran and Simon 1988), pigmented onychomatricoma (Wynes et al. 2015), and onychocytic matricoma (Perrin et al. 2012). Pigmented onychomycosis may also be a close mimic of longitudinal melanonychia due to a neoplasm. Finally, nail plate hemorrhage occasionally mimics a melanocytic proliferation. In some cases, the nail plate alone, sampled either during nail plate avulsion or in a nail clipping, can serve as a less invasive screening procedure for identifying the cause of nail plate discoloration. Of course, nail unit biopsy is often needed if melanin is identified, for confirmation and classification of the lesion responsible.

Histological Features in Nail Plate Samples

Melanin in the nail plate is usually observed as granular pigmentation of varying intensity. It can be very subtle in melanocytic activation, and one may need to utilize Fontana–Masson staining in some cases to highlight it (Fig. 10.1). Melanin

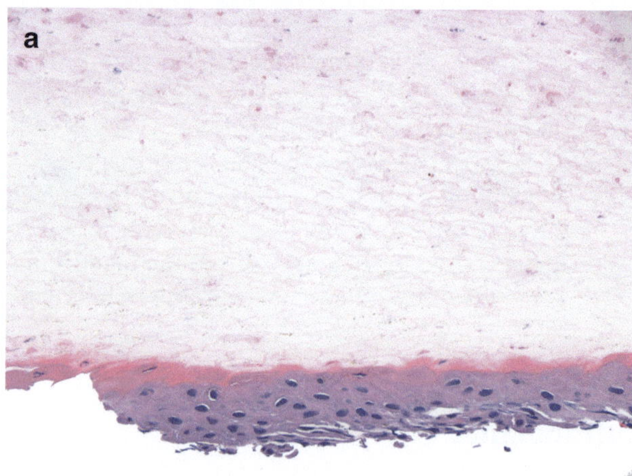

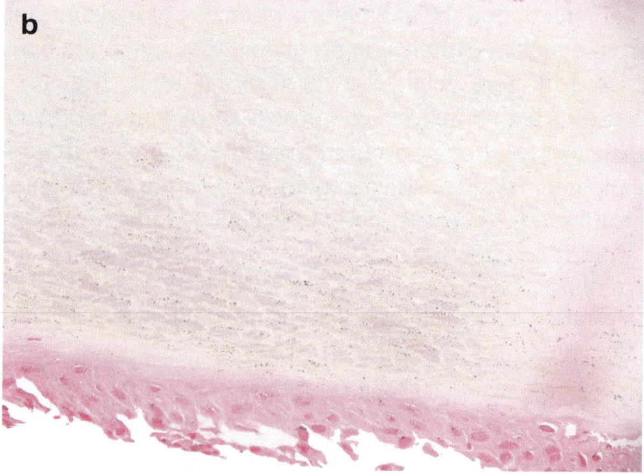

Fig. 10.1 Melanonychia in melanocytic activation. (**a**) Subtle fine melanin granules in H&E-stained sections of nail plate with attached nail bed epithelium. (**b**) Fontana–Masson staining of the same sections, highlighting melanin in the nail plate and epithelium

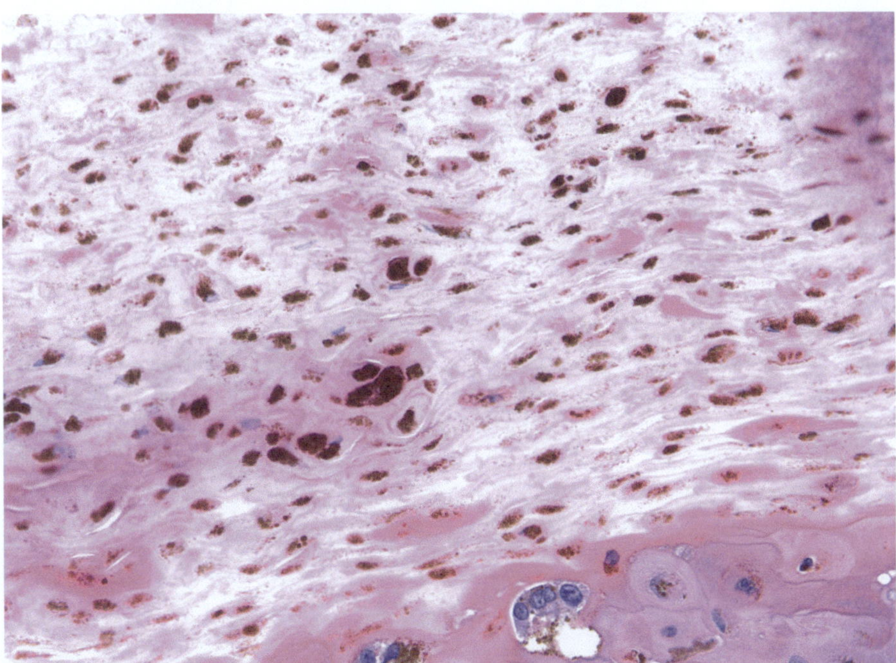

Fig. 10.2 Melanonychia in a nail unit melanoma. Irregular globules and granules of melanin in the nail plate, and atypical melanocytes in irregular array in the subjacent nail bed epithelium

pigmentation is usually somewhat regular/periodic, but can be irregular, including globules of pigment, more commonly in melanoma and on occasion in nevi, particularly in children (Fig. 10.2). Pigment that arises from the distal matrix, a common origin of pigmented lesions in the nail unit, is deposited in the lower two thirds of the plate, whereas more proximal lesions may occur in the upper third. Of course, lesions that involve the nail matrix more diffusely may involve the full thickness of the nail plate. This distribution of pigmentation can be observed dermoscopically in some cases if the nail plate is examined at its distal free edge, and histologically, including in nail plate samples (Fig. 10.3). When melanin is identified in the nail plate, it is frequently observed in any attached nail unit epithelium too (Fig. 10.1b). It is very important for a pathologist to pay close attention to the examination of this epithelium, which may be ample, as melanocytes may be present as well. These can also find their way into the nail plate proper, most commonly in melanoma, but in some nevi as well, particularly in children, as a function of the suprabasal scatter of melanocytes, singly and/or in nests (Ruben and McCalmont 2010; Boni et al. 2015). This is generally a worrisome feature in adults, especially if extensive (Fig. 10.4).

Pigmented onychomycosis arises from infection of the nail plate with dematiaceous fungi and molds (Perrin and Baran 1994; Finch et al. 2012). Common species are *Scytalidium*, *Scopulariopsis*, and *Trichophyton rubrum* var. *nigricans* and are a particularly common problem in tropical climates. The infection may take the form

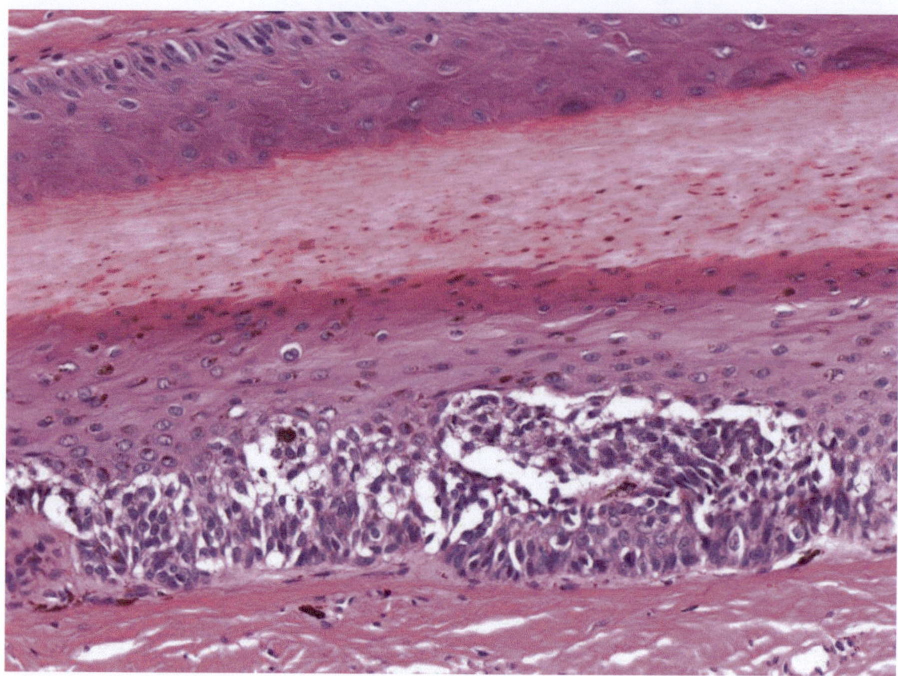

Fig. 10.3 Melanonychia in a nail nevus. Longitudinal nail unit biopsy demonstrating nests of melanocytes in the distal nail matrix, and melanin granules in the lower two-thirds of the nail plate

of superficial onychomycosis, dermatophytoma (in which the organisms are often loculated and form a mass under or within the nail plate) or other patterns in between (Fig. 10.5). The pigmentation within such organisms is melanin within their cell walls, and can also be confirmed as such by Fontana–Masson stain. One of the reasons it is important to submit the nail plate during nail unit biopsies for suspected melanonychia if removed is to avoid missing this cause of pigmentation (and hemorrhage, see below).

Nail unit hemorrhage can often be diagnosed clinically and via dermoscopy, but nail clippings or avulsions are commonly submitted as well in questionable cases. This is manifested as loculated hemorrhage, rather than the granular pigment of melanoma. It can be subungual, and/or intraungual and may be overt or very subtle, as tiny loculations. A modified benzidine stain can be used to identify the hemoglobins in subtle cases (Hafner et al. 1995) (Fig. 10.6). The commonly used stains for identifying hemosiderin in tissue, namely Perls' or Prussian blue, cannot be used in this setting, as the hemorrhage occurs in an avascular space, in which enzymes required to convert hemoglobin to hemosiderin are not accessible. As noted above, melanin can find its way into the nail plate as a result of melanocytic activation, and this can accompany inflammatory, infectious, neoplastic, and traumatic conditions. For example, a traumatic lesion containing hemorrhage may also contain melanin. Conversely, hemorrhage can occur secondarily in any of these settings as well. Therefore, if hemorrhage is found, the clinician must follow the nail outgrowth if

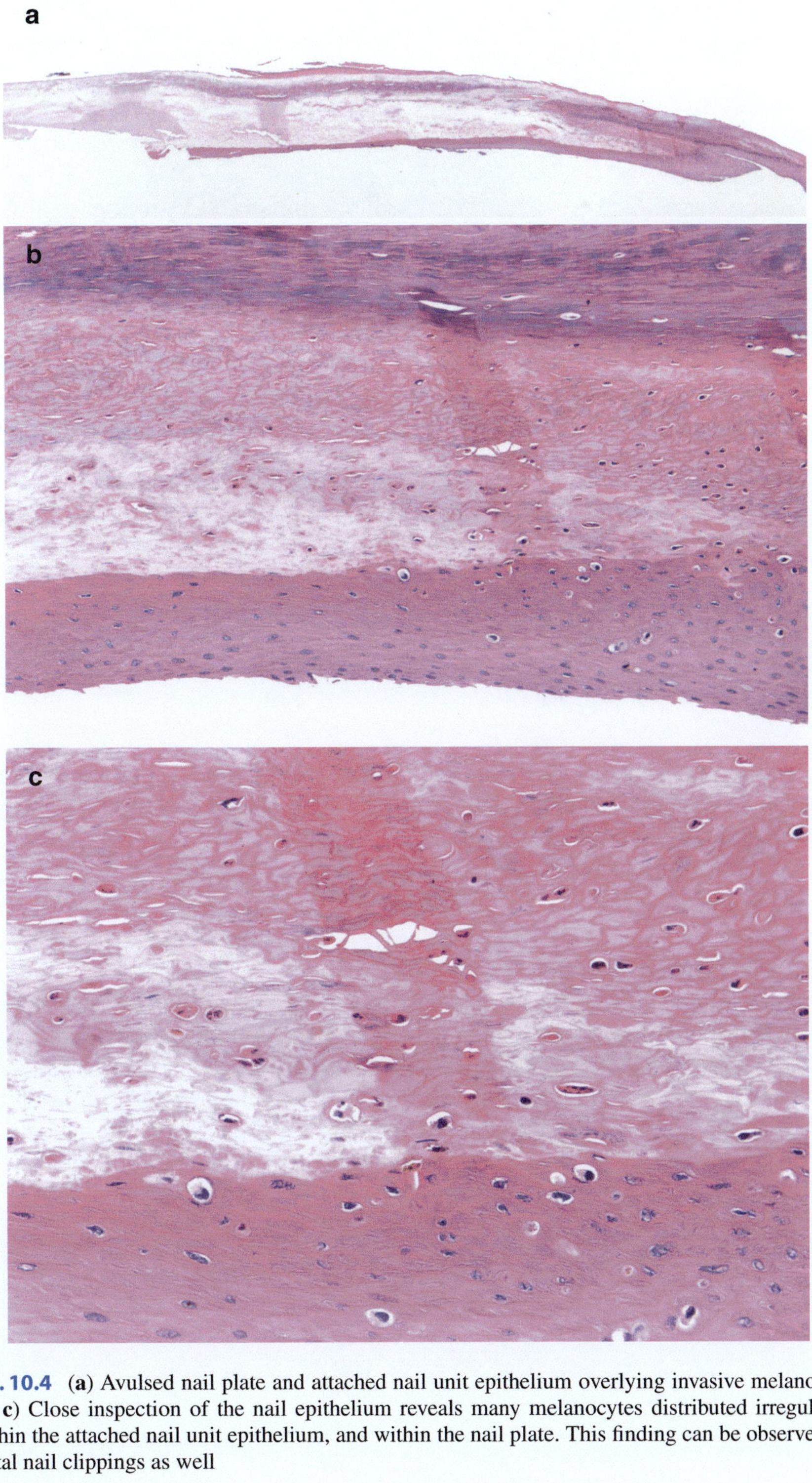

Fig. 10.4 (**a**) Avulsed nail plate and attached nail unit epithelium overlying invasive melanoma. (**b**, **c**) Close inspection of the nail epithelium reveals many melanocytes distributed irregularly within the attached nail unit epithelium, and within the nail plate. This finding can be observed in distal nail clippings as well

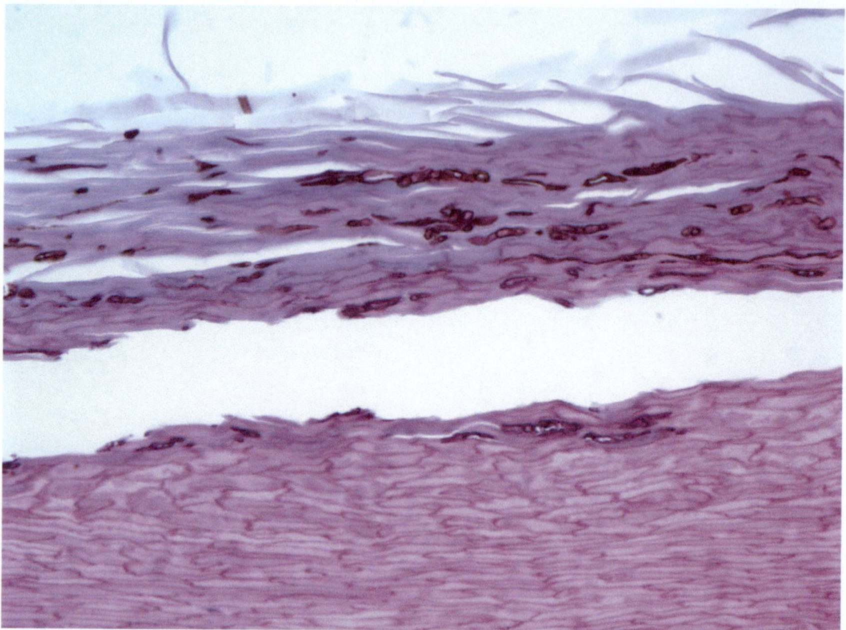

Fig. 10.5 Pigmented superficial onychomycosis. Numerous pigmented hyphae within the outer nail plate in a PAS-D stain. The melanin within the cell walls of such organisms can also be detected by Fontana–Masson stain

not avulsed, to ensure that the discoloration moves distally and resolves as expected. If melanin is identified, nail unit biopsy may be warranted to exclude a melanocytic or other neoplasm producing melanin.

Summary for the Clinician
Pigmentation of the nail plate may have many causes: melanocytic activation or proliferation, pigmented squamous cell carcinoma, pigmented onychomatricoma, onychocytic matricoma, pigmented onychomycosis, and nail plate hemorrhage. It is important to remember that nail sampling can be a useful screening tool in identifying the type of nail plate discoloration. If melanin, additional biopsy may be needed. Hemorrhage can occur secondarily in many conditions; thus, the clinician should ensure that this type of discoloration moves distally and resolves as expected to avoid overlooking other potential causes of the hemorrhage.

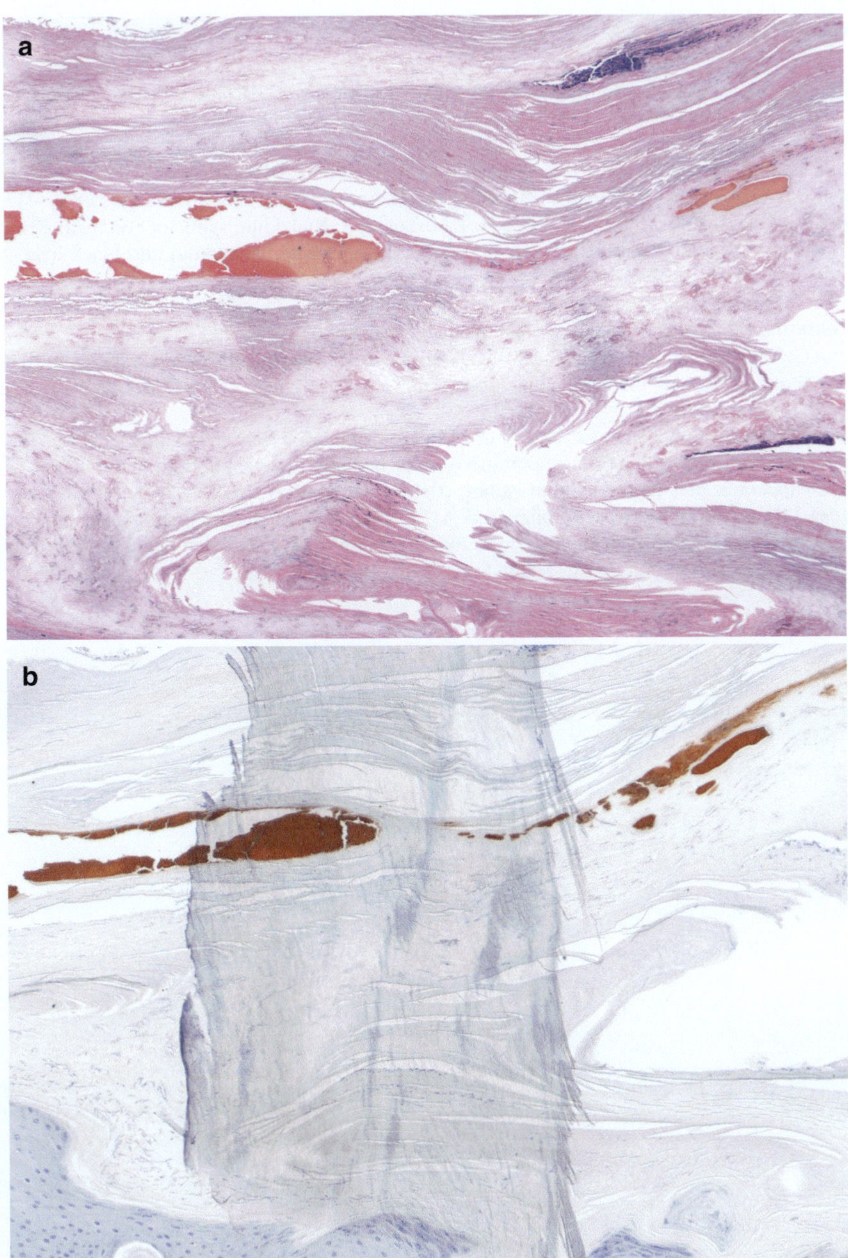

Fig. 10.6 Hemorrhage within the nail plate. (**a**) Loculated hemorrhage within a distorted nail plate. (**b**) The hemorrhage is highlighted by a modified benzidine stain

References

Baran R, Simon C. Longitudinal melanonychia: a symptom of Bowen's disease. J Am Acad Dermatol. 1988;18(6):1359–60.

Boni A, Chu EY, Rubin AI. Routine nail clipping leads to the diagnosis of amelanotic nail unit melanoma in a young construction worker. J Cutan Pathol. 2015;42(8):505–9.

Finch J, Arenas R, Baran R. Fungal melanonychia. J Am Acad Dermatol. 2012;66(5):830–41.

Hafner J, Haenseler E, Ossent P, Burg G, Panizzon RG. Benzidine stain for the histochemical detection of hemoglobin in splinter hemorrhage (subungual hematoma) and black heel. Am J Dermatopathol. 1995;17(4):362–7.

Perrin C, Baran R. Longitudinal melanonychia caused by trichophyton rubrum. Histochemical and ultrastructural study of two cases. J Am Acad Dermatol. 1994;31(2 Pt 2):311–6.

Perrin C, Cannata GE, Bossard C, Grill JM, Ambrossetti D, Michiels J-F. Onychocytic matricoma presenting as pachymelanonychia longitudinal. A new entity (report of five cases). Am J Dermatopathol. 2012;34(1):54–9.

Ruben BS. Pigmented lesions of the nail unit. Semin Cutan Med Surg. 2015;34(2):101–8.

Ruben BS, McCalmont TH. The importance of attached nail plate epithelium in the diagnosis of nail apparatus melanoma. J Cutan Pathol. 2010;37(10):1028–9. 1027.

Wynes J, Wanat KA, Huen A, Mlodzienski AJ, Rubin AI. Pigmented onychomatricoma: a rare pigmented nail unit tumor presenting as longitudinal melanonychia that has potential for misdiagnosis as melanoma. J Foot Ankle Surg. 2015;54(4):723–5.

Biopsy

11

Lucy Chen, Giselle Prado, and Martin Zaiac

> **Key Features**
> - Melanonychia that is suspicious for melanoma should be biopsied to provide a histopathological diagnosis of the lesion.
> - A detailed understanding of the anatomy of the nail unit and the various nail biopsy techniques results in optimal outcomes in both function and aesthetic appearance.
> - Before biopsy, it is imperative to perform a complete assessment of the patient, a detailed physical examination of the nail unit, and dermoscopic inspection of the nail plate, proximal nail fold, and free edge.
> - The key decision when executing nail biopsy is selecting the best technique based on the location, width, and index of suspicion.
> - The most pertinent complication after nail surgery is nail dystrophy due to damage to the proximal nail matrix.

L. Chen, MD (✉)
Department of Dermatology and Cutaneous Surgery,
University of Miami, 1600 NW 10th Ave, Miami, FL 33136, United States
e-mail: lucychendermatology@gmail.com

G. Prado, BS
Herbert Wertheim College of Medicine, Florida International University, 11200 SW 8 St., Miami, FL 33199, United States

M. Zaiac, MD
Director Greater Miami Skin and Laser Center,
Mount Sinai Medical Center, 4308 Alton Road, Suite 750,
Miami Beach, FL 33140, United States

© Springer International Publishing Switzerland 2017
N. Di Chiacchio, A. Tosti (eds.), *Melanonychias*,
DOI 10.1007/978-3-319-44993-7_11

Introduction

Although some melanocytic lesions of the nail unit can be confidently diagnosed on the basis of clinical presentation and dermoscopy alone, some melanonychia may be indicative of underlying melanomas rather than benign tumors. It has been shown that accuracy of the diagnosis of nail melanoma, especially thin tumors, by dermatologists is low, even among nail experts (Di Chiacchio et al. 2010). Melanonychia in which melanoma is suspected should be biopsied by a dermatological surgeon to provide a histopathological diagnosis of the lesion. The poor prognosis associated with a delayed diagnosis of nail apparatus melanoma portends a need for heightened vigilance.

Indications for Biopsy

Given the multitude of possible etiologies, dermatologists should be aware of definitive indications for biopsying longitudinal melanonychia. Certainly, the first task is to differentiate melanonychia as either melanocytic or nonmelanocytic in origin. Nonmelanic lesions that appear melanocytic, such as subungual hemorrhage and exogenous toxins, can mimic a malignant lesion. Melanonychia more commonly arises because of nail matrix melanocyte activation, nail matrix melanocyte proliferation, or invasion by melanin-producing pathogens than malignancy. Dermoscopy can help to differentiate these causes, but ultimately biopsy may be necessary (Di Chiacchio et al. 2013; Ronger et al. 2002).

A detailed understanding of the anatomy of the nail unit and the various nail biopsy techniques available to the dermatological surgeon results in optimal outcomes in both function and aesthetic appearance. The physician should be alerted to the possibility of malignancy based on a detailed history, physical examination of the skin and mucous membranes, and dermoscopic evaluation of the nail unit (Table 11.1).

Table 11.1 Indications for the biopsy of longitudinal melanonychia to rule out melanoma

1. Isolated band on a single band that develops between the fourth and sixth decade of life
2. Abrupt growth of or change in the lesion
3. Pigmentation that begins after a history of digital trauma and in which subungual hematoma has been ruled out
4. Acquired pigmentation in a person with a personal history of melanoma
5. Nail pigmentation that has resulted in nail destruction or dystrophy
6. The presence of Hutchinson's sign – pigmentation present on the periungual skin, including at the cuticle or hyponychium
7. Dermoscopically worrisome pattern of the nail plate

Adapted from Braun et al. (2007)

Anatomy of the Nail Unit

The critical structures of the nail unit are the nail matrix, nail bed, proximal and lateral nail folds, hyponychium, and nail plate. The nail matrix is the center from which matrical keratinocytes generate the nail plate. Its distal end can be visualized as the lunula, the half-moon structure, at the cuticle of the proximal nail fold. The distal nail matrix generates the ventral nail plate, whereas the proximal nail matrix forms the dorsal nail plate. Any damage to the nail matrix has the ability to irreversibly scar the nail. The nail bed is attached underneath the nail plate by tight cellular adhesions. There is no subcutaneous tissue; thus, a full-thickness biopsy or excision should reach the periosteum.

Hemostasis and Anesthesia

Blood flow to the nail is supplied by lateral digital arteries that course along the sides of the digit and form distal superficial branches. For hand surgery, a sterile glove with the fingertip cut out and rolled back can be used for the dual function of hemostasis and sterility (Harrington et al. 2004). Alternatively, hemostasis can be achieved by applying gentle pressure to the lateral sides of the digit by an assistant. It is crucial to release the glove or tourniquet every 15–20 min to avoid tissue ischemia.

Innervation to the nail unit is supplied by cutaneous sensory nerves that run in parallel with the blood vessels. Adequate anesthesia is crucial to this procedure owing to patient apprehension and sensitivity to pain of the nail unit. The two most common options for anesthesia are the digital ring block or the wing block (Rich 2001). The digital ring block introduces lidocaine injections on either side of the base of the digit. The wing block introduces anesthesia to the proximal and lateral nail folds in smaller volumes and has a more rapid onset of action than the digital block. Small volumes (less than 1.0 mL) should be injected at any given site to reduce the risk of vasospasm or vessel tamponade. There are numerous reviews that detail the safe use of lidocaine with epinephrine for digital blocks, with no reports of digital necrosis from commercial lidocaine with epinephrine (Krunic et al. 2004; Wilhelmi et al. 2001). For less pain and discomfort with subcutaneous injection, this author prefers to dilute 3 mL of 1% lidocaine with 1:100,000 epinephrine in 30 mL of bacteriostatic 0.9% sodium chloride in a 1:10 ratio (Zaiac et al. 2012). In our experience, the wing block technique is sufficient anesthesia during the biopsy of melanonychia.

Preoperative Preparation

Before biopsy, a detailed medical history must be obtained from the patient to assess operative bleeding risk and the likelihood of complications. Risk factors such as smoking, diabetes, peripheral vascular disease, Raynaud's phenomenon, immunocompromised states, prosthetic joints or heart valves, connective tissue disease and the use of anticoagulation therapies confer increased risk of developing complications (Rich 2001; Weiss and Zaiac 2015). Smoking cessation should be advised several weeks before the procedure if possible. Prophylactic antibiotics are not necessary for nail biopsy unless the procedure carries a high risk of infection (Wright et al. 2008). Physical examination should include palpation of distal pulses and any signs of cutaneous infection or impaired perfusion should be noted. The procedure should be explained to the patient with a discussion of the possible complications, benefits of surgery, and associated risks, including permanent nail dystrophy. A signed written informed consent form should be obtained.

Preoperative photography is highly recommended. In our practice, we utilize high-quality digital dermoscopy and keep these photographs as part of the medical record. Nail plate dermoscopy is easy to capture and is imperative for establishing indications for biopsy. If melanonychia lacks malignant features under dermoscopy, photographs can be taken to monitor for interval change.

The patient should be positioned lying or sitting comfortable with the limb to be biopsied supported in a neutral position. The dorsal aspect of the limb should be exposed to allow visualization of the nail. The affected hand or foot should be cleansed with chlorhexidine or equivalent surgical soap and sterilely draped.

Procedure

Once the decision has been made to biopsy a patient with melanonychia, careful planning maximizes the sampled specimen while minimizing permanent nail deformity. Keeping in mind the location of the area of melanonychia to be biopsied and the degree of suspicion for invasive disease help the dermatological surgeon to choose the best biopsy technique. The nail matrix, which contains the origin of the pigment, must be adequately sampled. Nail matrix biopsy is associated with the highest risk of scarring compared with other nail unit locations. Distal matrix biopsy is preferred over proximal biopsy because any resulting defect can be hidden in the ventral surface of the nail plate.

Dermoscopic examination of the free edge of the nail can give a clue to the site of pigmentation origin in vivo. Pigment on the upper nail plate indicates that it originates in the proximal matrix, whereas if only the lower part of the nail plate has pigment, the distal matrix is the source (Fig. 11.1). This technique correlates accurately with nail plate clipping and Fontana–Masson staining and is quick and more cost-effective (Braun et al. 2006). If the nail fold demonstrates Hutchinson's sign, submitting a shave biopsy of this pigmented area may help to make the diagnosis. Certainly, other conditions with pseudo-Hutchinson's sign must be excluded (Baran and Kechijian 1996).

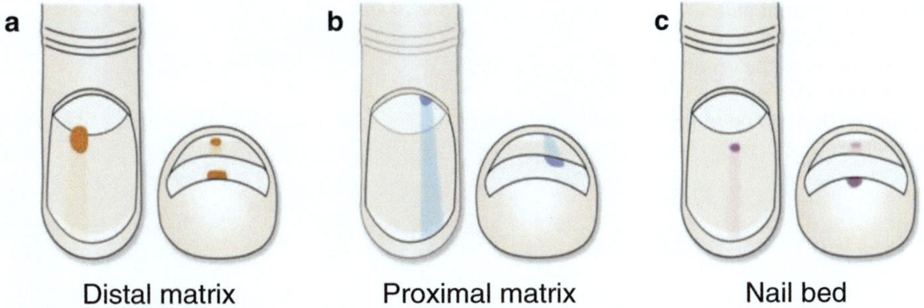

Fig. 11.1 Location of the origin of melanonychia pigment according to the nail plate and free edge view. (**a**) Distal matrix pigmentation is visible on the lower part of the free edge of the nail. (**b**) Proximal matrix pigmentation is seen on the upper part of the free edge. (**c**) Nail bed pigmentation is appreciated in the lowest part of the free edge

Exposure and Visualization of the Nail Matrix

Following adequate anesthesia, two tangential parallel incisions are made at the lateral aspects of the proximal nail fold. A nail elevator can be carefully inserted to undermine the nail fold away from the underlying nail matrix. The proximal nail fold is then reflected back by skin hooks or sutures to reveal the proximal nail plate and matrix.

The author uses intraoperative dermoscopy to visualize the exposed matrix and nail bed. The instrument should be viewed in noncontact mode to avoid contamination of the surgical field. The presence of an irregular dermoscopic pattern consisting of longitudinal lines of irregular colors and thicknesses has been observed in greater frequency in nail melanoma compared with benign melanocytic hyperplasia or nevi (Hirata et al. 2011).

Complete or Partial Nail Avulsion

The conventional approach to nail biopsy was to completely avulse the entire nail plate, thus allowing direct visualization of the nail unit. However, newer methods support the use of less invasive and destructive techniques whenever possible (Collins et al. 2008).

Partial proximal nail plate avulsion is a technique well-suited to melanonychia biopsy (Collins et al. 2008). First, the proximal nail fold should be reflected back to visualize the matrix, as described above. Starting at one lateral edge, approximately half-way between the cuticle and free distal edge, the nail plate is cut transversely with an English nail splitter. The nail piece is reflected laterally to one side to expose the matrix, similar to opening the hood of a car (Fig. 11.2).

Another partial nail biopsy technique, the "submarine hatch" can be used for small lesions less than 3 mm wide and allows for adequate exposure of the nail matrix (Zaiac et al. 2014). A standard 5-mm punch is applied obliquely to the nail

Fig. 11.2 Partial nail avulsion allows for visualization of the origin of pigmentation without complete destruction of the nail plate

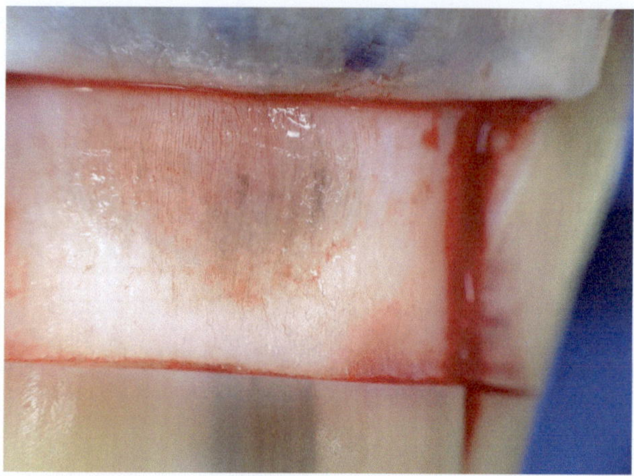

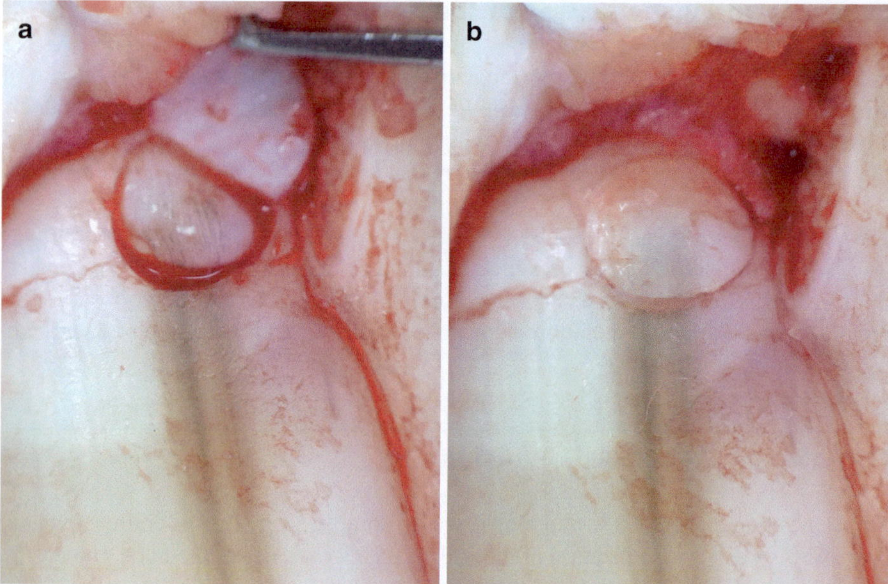

Fig. 11.3 The submarine hatch: the nail plate is hinged open by applying oblique pressure with a punch tool. (**a**) The proximal nail matrix is exposed and a punch biopsy of suspicious pigmentation can be performed. (**b**) Exposed nail plate is moved back into place and secured with cyanoacrylate adhesive to act as a biological dressing

plate and gently twisted to allow the plate to hinge open. The nail plate remains hinged open while the underlying matrix specimen is obtained using the punch method (Fig. 11.3). Hemostasis can be achieved by pressure and the plate is re-glued with ethyl cyanoacrylate.

Alternatively, the trap-door avulsion technique can be used for lesions greater than 3 mm wide (Fig. 11.4). This technique is useful for lesions originating in the

Fig. 11.4 After trap door avulsion of the nail plate, the nail matrix specimen is sampled with a no. 15 blade in (**a**) proximal to (**b**) distal direction. Normal saline infiltration by injection creates tissue edema to facilitate a tangential shave biopsy of the proximal nail matrix

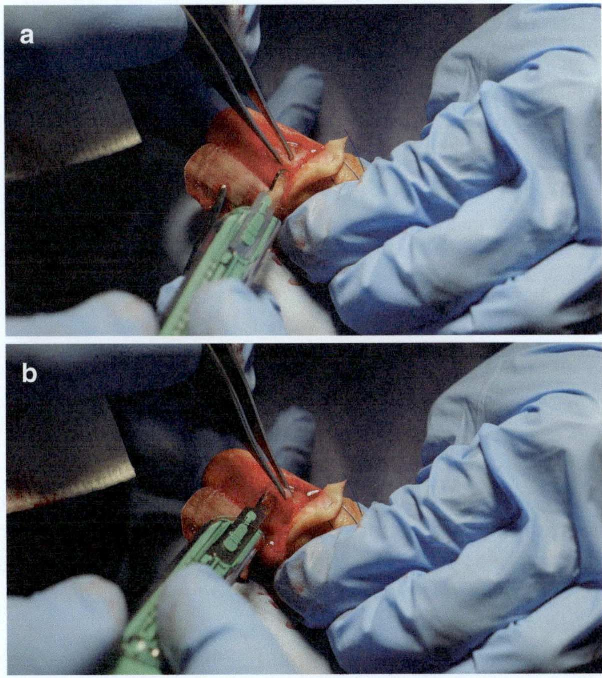

distal matrix and can be achieved without reflecting back the proximal nail fold (Collins et al. 2008).

Unless there is a frank melanoma, which would warrant complete plate removal, it is the author's opinion that partial nail avulsion is sufficient for the biopsy of melanonychia. Furthermore, remaining pigmentation on the distal nail plate acts as a guide to the best location to take a biopsy, especially when the matrix lacks gross pigmentation.

Tangential Shave Nail Matrix Biopsy

For melanonychia with pigmentation greater than 3 mm, or located near the midline, the tangential shave biopsy of the nail matrix produces a reliable biopsy sample (Haneke and Baran 2001; Di Chiacchio et al. 2012; Richert et al. 2013). In fact, some authors state that this technique is the best for tissue-sparing and yields a minimal risk of scarring (Haneke 2011).

After proximal nail plate avulsion, the matrix is carefully examined to locate the origin of pigmentation. The remaining band on the distal nail plate can be used as a guide. In addition, intraoperative dermoscopy directly on the matrix can identify the most suspicious foci of pigmentation. At this point, we inject a small amount of 0.9% sodium chloride to elevate the matrix of interest (Fig. 11.5). This tissue edema guides a more precise biopsy technique. Then, a no. 15 blade

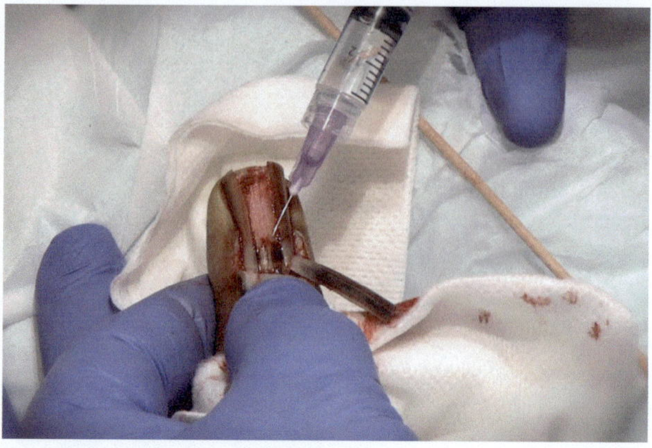

Fig. 11.5 Normal saline infiltration by injection creates tissue edema to facilitate a tangential shave biopsy of the proximal nail matrix

is used to score 1- to 2-mm margins around the lesion (Fig. 11.4). By holding the blade parallel to the matrix, the specimen is tangentially excised with sawing motions back and forth. Care should be taken to handle the specimen without forceps to avoid tissue trauma. The shave specimen should be marked, fixed, and placed on filter paper to ensure that the matrix specimen will lay flat without curling (Jellinek 2007).

The avulsed nail plate should be handled gently, because it can be replaced after surgery to act as a natural protective dressing and reduce postoperative complications and morbidity. To facilitate the replacement of the nail plate after surgery, the nail plate can be trimmed by 1–2 mm at the lateral edge to reduce embedding with postoperative edema (Collins et al. 2008). There are weak adhesions between the avulsed nail plate and the bed; thus, as the new nail plate grows, the avulsed plate may undergo onychomadesis. The reflected nail plate is laid back into place and can be sutured to the lateral nail fold with 3-0 non-absorbable nylon sutures. The proximal nail fold incisions are also sutured with non-absorbable sutures or brought together with skin adhesive.

Three-Millimeter Punch Biopsy Excision

For bands of melanonychia less than 3 mm in width, a punch biopsy without nail avulsion can yield sufficient tissue to make a histological diagnosis. Using a 3-mm punch biopsy for lesions wider than 3 mm may result in a false-negative result. Multiple punch biopsies performed to sample a wide band are at an even higher risk for causing nail dystrophy and may not adequately sample the entire lesion.

It is imperative to first identify the pigmented band's origin at the proximal nail plate. It is our preference to use the "submarine hatch" technique so that the nail plate can easily be retained to act as a biological dressing (Fig. 11.3). Once visualized, a 3-mm punch is introduced through the matrix down to the periosteum. Forceps should be avoided to reduce the risk for a crushing injury to the fragile specimen. Rather, sharp-tipped scissors are used to carefully dissect around and snip out the tissue. The vault of the punch instrument should always be examined for any adhered pieces of nail plate. Some authors advise submitting these in separately labeled formalin jars to avoid missed sections during processing (Jellinek 2007). The remaining defect can be left to heal with the nail plate replaced and dressed with skin adhesives.

The punch biopsy technique can also be performed without nail plate avulsion. To facilitate the removal of biopsy tissue, a "double punch" method can be employed. A larger 6-mm punch diameter can be used to cut through the nail plate and then a smaller 3-mm punch is inserted within to allow easier access to the biopsy material (Krull 2001a). The avulsed nail plate can be replaced back into the defect and glued with ethyl cyanoacrylate.

It has been our experience that defects less than 3 mm heal without scarring and we infrequently perform matrical closures for defects greater than this size.

If the biopsy site involves the proximal matrix, the defect should be closed to minimize nail injury and scarring. Some authors propose closing the defect if the proximal 10–20% of the matrix is involved (Krull 2001a).

Lateral Longitudinal Nail Biopsy or Excision

This technique is useful for pigmentation located in the lateral one-third of the nail plate (Krull 2001b). The lateral portion of the nail unit is excised en bloc including the proximal nail fold, lateral nail fold, nail matrix, nail plate, and hyponychium. A scalpel cut is made 1–2 mm medial to the pigmentation, deep through the nail plate, and the tissue piece is loosened from the underlying periosteum. The tissue specimen is removed entirely like a sliver of pie and submitted for histopathology. The fixed tissue should be cut longitudinally, not "bread-loafed."

Before closure, remaining small matricial fragments must be removed to avoid spicules or cyst formation. The defect can be closed by bringing together the proximal nail fold to the lateral nail fold, and the remaining nail plate to the lateral nail fold using interrupted absorbable sutures. Alternatively, the defect may be left to heal by secondary intention.

Longitudinal Matrix Excision

This technique can be utilized when a shave or punch biopsy is not adequate for sampling the pigment in question or when a full-thickness biopsy is desired owing to concern regarding an invasive melanoma. After visualization of the nail matrix by partial nail plate avulsion, a longitudinal elliptical excision is made with 1- to 2-mm margins at the origin of the melanonychia. Innovative flap reconstruction techniques reduce the occurrence of thin or split nail (Collins et al. 2010).

Broad Bands of Longitudinal Melanonychia

For bands between 3 and 6 mm or when there is diffuse melanonychia, broader sampling of the pigmentation is required. A transverse matrix biopsy can be employed (Braun et al. 2007). This type of biopsy is technically demanding as the incision should match the curvature of the lunula and extend to the periosteum. The edges of the matrix must be carefully re-approximated after undermining of the surrounding tissue. Alternatively, if there is a high index of suspicion for invasive melanoma, en bloc excision of all nail tissue can be carried out.

Submitting the Specimen

It imperative to provide as much supplementary information as possible to the pathologist when submitting a nail specimen. It is our practice to submit the specimen on a labeled paper with "proximal" and "distal" orientation clearly marked. The requisition sheet also explicitly details the components of submission, drawing of the nail apparatus with the exact location of the band of melanonychia, the site of biopsy, and the technique used (for example, "tangential shave biopsy of the distal matrix of mid-line melanonychia from the second digit"). The specimen is submitted in formalin in a cassette, along with the detailed requisition sheet (Fig. 11.6).

Postprocedural Care

After the procedure, the surgical site must have complete hemostasis. Although some surgeons are proponents of hemostatic gelatin sponges (i.e., Gelfoam), our experience has shown more postoperative inflammation with these measures. The

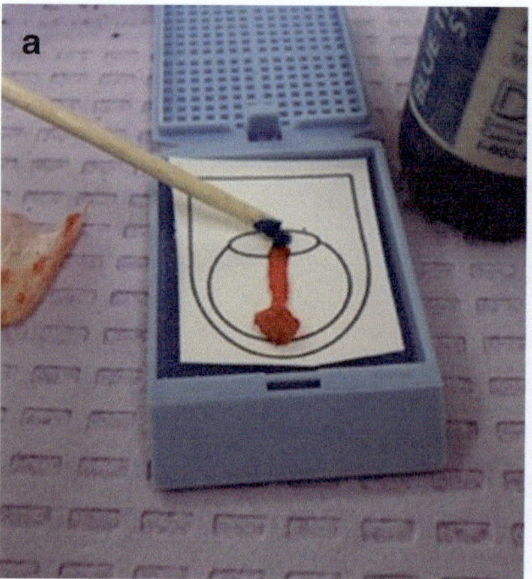
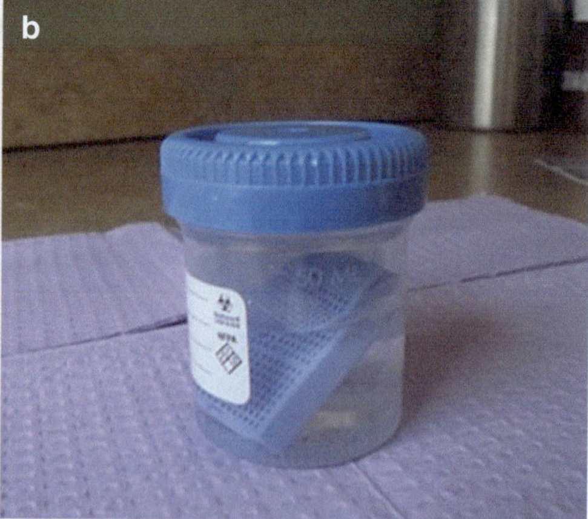

Fig. 11.6 (**a**) The sampled specimen is submitted with a marked drawing and enclosed in a cassette. (**b**) The cassette is submitted in a formalin bottle with the appropriate requisition form (Images courtesy of Drs Curtis Thompson and Phoebe Rich)

patient should be observed for 15 min to assess for bleeding and to mitigate a potential vasovagal response.

The site should be irrigated with normal saline and a layer of antibiotic ointment should be applied. A nonstick dressing such as petrolatum-impregnated gauze or Telfa should cover the surgical site. The bandage should be loose to account for postoperative edema and to avoid strangulation of the digit. The bandage should be changed every 24 h and the wound cleansed with soap and water before applying a new bandage. Pain control can be achieved with acetaminophen instead of nonsteroidal anti-inflammatory medications to maintain platelet function. Opiates may be necessary for the short-term control of pain. Sutures can be removed after 10–14 days.

Potential Complications

Biopsy of the nail unit is well tolerated and serious complications rarely occur (Moossavi and Scher 2001). The most common adverse outcomes include dystrophy of the nail plate due to damage of the nail matrix and split nail. Scarring at the proximal nail fold results in dorsal pterygium, whereas scarring of the nail bed can result in onycholysis due to scarring of the nail bed. Infections and subungual hematomas are uncommon complications. Postoperative oral antibiotics for the prevention of surgical site infections are only indicated for certain high-risk individuals. One study found that 47% of patients go on to develop dysesthesia, although most experience resolution within 6–12 months (Walsh et al. 2009).

> **Summary for the Clinician**
> Biopsy of melanonychia is not a common procedure for the practicing dermatologist, but with enough training and expertise in the anatomy of the nail unit, any dermatologist can comfortably perform this procedure. Dermatologists should keep in mind the procedures outlined in this chapter to effectively perform a nail biopsy of melanonychia where melanoma is suspected.

References

Baran R, Kechijian P. Hutchinson's sign: a reappraisal. J Am Acad Dermatol. 1996;34(1):87–90.

Braun RP, Baran R, Saurat JH, Thomas L. Surgical pearl: dermoscopy of the free edge of the nail to determine the level of nail plate pigmentation and the location of its probable origin in the proximal or distal nail matrix. J Am Acad Dermatol. 2006;55(3):512–3.

Braun RP, Baran R, Le Gal FA, Dalle S, Ronger S, Pandolfi R, et al. Diagnosis and management of nail pigmentations. J Am Acad Dermatol. 2007;56(5):835–47.

Collins SC, Cordova K, Jellinek NJ. Alternatives to complete nail plate avulsion. J Am Acad Dermatol. 2008;59(4):619–26.

Collins SC, Cordova KB, Jellinek NJ. Midline/paramedian longitudinal matrix excision with flap reconstruction: alternative surgical techniques for evaluation of longitudinal melanonychia. J Am Acad Dermatol. 2010;62(4):627–36.

Di Chiacchio N, Hirata SH, Enokihara MY, Michalany NS, Fabbrocini G, Tosti A. Dermatologists' accuracy in early diagnosis of melanoma of the nail matrix. Arch Dermatol. 2010;146(4):382–7.

Di Chiacchio N, Loureiro WR, Michalany NS, Kezam Gabriel FV. Tangential biopsy thickness versus lesion depth in longitudinal melanonychia: a pilot study. Dermatol Res Pract. 2012;2012:353864.

Di Chiacchio ND, Farias DC, Piraccini BM, Hirata SH, Richert B, Zaiac M, et al. Consensus on melanonychia nail plate dermoscopy. An Bras Dermatol. 2013;88(2):309–13.

Haneke E. Advanced nail surgery. J Cutan Aesthet Surg. 2011;4(3):167–75.

Haneke E, Baran R. Longitudinal melanonychia. Dermatol Surg. 2001;27(6):580–4.

Harrington AC, Cheyney JM, Kinsley-Scott T, Willard RJ. A novel digital tourniquet using a sterile glove and hemostat. Dermatol Surg. 2004;30(7):1065–7.

Hirata SH, Yamada S, Enokihara MY, Di Chiacchio N, de Almeida FA, Enokihara MM, et al. Patterns of nail matrix and bed of longitudinal melanonychia by intraoperative dermatoscopy. J Am Acad Dermatol. 2011;65(2):297–303.

Jellinek N. Nail matrix biopsy of longitudinal melanonychia: diagnostic algorithm including the matrix shave biopsy. J Am Acad Dermatol. 2007;56(5):803–10.

Krull EA. Biopsy techniques. In: Krull EA, Zook E, Baran R, Haneke E, editors. Nail surgery: a text and atlas. Philadelphia: Lippincott Williams & Wilkins; 2001a. p. 55–81.

Krull EA. Longitudinal melanonychia. In: Krull EA, Zook E, Baran R, Haneke E, editors. Nail surgery: a text and atlas. Philadelphia: Lippincott Williams & Wilkins; 2001b. p. 239–74.

Krunic AL, Wang LC, Soltani K, Weitzul S, Taylor RS. Digital anesthesia with epinephrine: an old myth revisited. J Am Acad Dermatol. 2004;51(5):755–9.

Moossavi M, Scher RK. Complications of nail surgery: a review of the literature. Dermatol Surg. 2001;27(3):225–8.

Rich P. Nail biopsy: indications and methods. Dermatol Surg. 2001;27(3):229–34.

Richert B, Theunis A, Norrenberg S, Andre J. Tangential excision of pigmented nail matrix lesions responsible for longitudinal melanonychia: evaluation of the technique on a series of 30 patients. J Am Acad Dermatol. 2013;69(1):96–104.

Ronger S, Touzet S, Ligeron C, Balme B, Viallard AM, Barrut D, et al. Dermoscopic examination of nail pigmentation. Arch Dermatol. 2002;138(10):1327–33.

Walsh ML, Shipley DV, de Berker DA. Survey of patients' experiences after nail surgery. Clin Exp Dermatol. 2009;34(5):e154–6.

Weiss J, Zaiac MN. Best way to remove a subungual tumor. Dermatol Clin. 2015;33(2):283–7.

Wilhelmi BJ, Blackwell SJ, Miller JH, Mancoll JS, Dardano T, Tran A, et al. Do not use epinephrine in digital blocks: myth or truth? Plast Reconstr Surg. 2001;107(2):393–7.

Wright TI, Baddour LM, Berbari EF, Roenigk RK, Phillips PK, Jacobs MA, et al. Antibiotic prophylaxis in dermatologic surgery: advisory statement 2008. J Am Acad Dermatol. 2008;59(3):464–73.

Zaiac M, Aguilera SB, Zaulyanov-Scanlan L, Caperton C, Chimento S. Virtually painless local anesthesia: diluted lidocaine proves to be superior to buffered lidocaine for subcutaneous infiltration. J Drugs Dermatol. 2012;11(10):e39–42.

Zaiac MN, Norton ES, Tosti A. The "submarine hatch" nail bed biopsy. J Am Acad Dermatol. 2014;70(6):e127–8.

Histopathological Analysis

12

Nilceo S. Michalany, Maria Victoria Suarez Restrepo, and Leandro Fonseca Noriega

> **Key Features**
> - Histological examination is considered the gold standard for the diagnosis of melanonychia.
> - Melanocytic lesions of the nail matrix can be caused by melanocytic activation (hypermelanosis) or by melanocytic proliferation (nevus or lentigo [benign] or melanoma [malignant]).
> - Immunohistochemistry techniques can be helpful in distinguishing malignant lesions from benign.

Introduction

Most cases of melanonychia result from benign diseases, which are mainly represented by melanocytic activation, lentigo, and nevus. These three pathological conditions can be further divided – according to their basic histological findings – into two large groups: (1) increased melanin without increased melanocytes, and (2) increased melanocytes. The first group is represented by melanocytic activation or hypermelanosis. The second group is characterized by benign melanocytic proliferation and can be subdivided into lentigo and nevus, according to the arrangement of melanocytes. Malignant melanocytic proliferation is represented by in situ or invasive melanoma (Ruben 2015; André et al. 2013; Fernandez-Flores et al. 2014).

N.S. Michalany, MD
Departamento de Dermatologia, da Universidade Federal de, São Paulo, Brazil

M.V. Suarez Restrepo, MD (✉) • L.F. Noriega, MD
Departamento de Dermatologia, Hospital do Servidor Publico Municipal, São Paulo, Brazil
e-mail: mariavsuarez@hotmail.com

© Springer International Publishing Switzerland 2017
N. Di Chiacchio, A. Tosti (eds.), *Melanonychias*,
DOI 10.1007/978-3-319-44993-7_12

Nonmelanocytic lesions can also cause pigmentary changes of the nail and should be included in the differential diagnoses, which include pigmented onychomycosis, subungual hematoma, pigmented keratinocytic or fibroepithelial proliferations, such as onychomatricoma, onychocytic matricoma, and squamous cell carcinoma in situ (Ruben 2015; Fernandez-Flores et al. 2014).

The clinical and dermoscopic features of nail apparatus lesions may be similar, making differential diagnosis complex. Therefore, histopathology is considered the gold standard diagnostic method, particularly in ambiguous cases. In such situations, immunohistochemistry techniques can help, as a complementary tool (Ruben 2015).

The anatomy of the nail unit is unique and it is important to remember certain concepts before exploring the histological features of melanonychia. In fact, under the nail matrix and nail bed there is a mesenchymal tissue called the onychodermis, which is typically devoid of stratum granulosum. Additionally, in this location, the subcutaneous fat is very thin or attenuated (André et al. 2013; Fernandez-Flores et al. 2014; Shin and Jang 2014). It is important to consider that the number of melanocytes is lower in the nail unit than in the rest of the skin, although the highest density of melanocytes in the nail unit is found in the nail matrix (André et al. 2013; Fernandez-Flores et al. 2014). In the proximal matrix, most melanocytes are inactive and do not produce any pigment (André et al. 2013; Fernandez-Flores et al. 2014). In the distal matrix, however, 50% are inactive and 50% active; in the nail bed, they are very rare and all of them dormant (André et al. 2013). In the proximal matrix, it is usual to find melanocytes located at the suprabasal layer (André et al. 2013; Fernandez-Flores et al. 2014; Shin and Jang 2014).

Being familiar with the anatomical peculiarities of the nail unit and its respective histological findings is essential for adequate interpretation (Ruben 2015; André et al. 2013; Fernandez-Flores et al. 2014).

Melanocytic Activation

Melanocytic activation is, by definition, an increase in melanin without augmentation of melanocyte density (Ruben 2015; André et al. 2013). It is also called hypermelanosis, functional melanonychia, and melanotic macule (Ruben 2015; André et al. 2013). Histologically, there is an increase in the pigment in the cytoplasm of some melanocytes, showing pigmented dendrites (André et al. 2013; Fernandez-Flores et al. 2014). Also, it is possible to observe pigmented keratinocytes and melanocytes can be found at a suprabasal location (André et al. 2013; Fernandez-Flores et al. 2014). For the pathologist, it is impossible to establish the origin of the melanocytic activation, except in the case of pigmented onychomycosis or Bowen's disease (André et al. 2013). If the pigment is barely visible, Fontana–Masson staining shows a few melanophages in the superficial dermis (Fig. 12.1) (André et al. 2013).

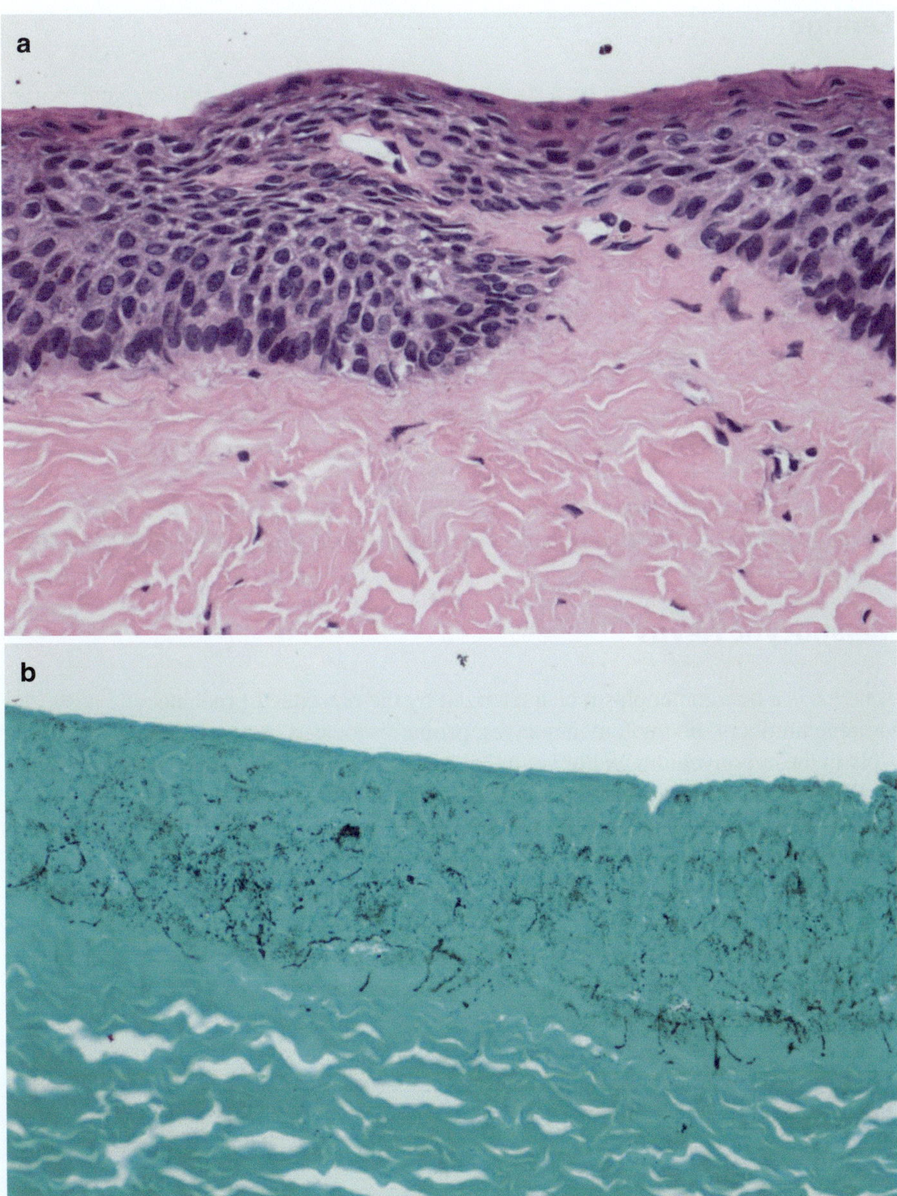

Fig. 12.1 (**a**) Melanocytic activation (hypermelanosis) showing melanocytic pigmentation of the matrix epithelium with no increase in the melanocytic density (H&E, ×200). (**b**) Fontana–Masson stain highlighting the melanocytic pigmentation of the matrix epithelium and active dendritic melanocytes (×200)

Lentigo

This entity is characterized by a slight-to-moderate increase in non-atypical – often dendritic – melanocytes in the nail matrix or nail bed, which remain arranged in individual units and are mainly located in the basal layer (Ruben 2015; André et al. 2013; Fernandez-Flores et al. 2014).

The density of matrix melanocytes ranges from 10 to 31 per millimeter and may be associated with melanophages (Ruben 2015; Amin et al. 2008). Mild atypia may occur. Mild and focal pagetoid spread, caused by non-atypical cells is rarely observed (André et al. 2013; Fernandez-Flores et al. 2014).

Unlike early melanoma, underlying stromal inflammatory infiltrate is usually absent (Fernandez-Flores et al. 2014).

When there is pronounced pigmentation of the background of keratinocytes, immunohistochemistry staining methods help to distinguish constituent melanocytes. Melan-A is useful, but may overestimate the melanocytic density. Microphthalmia transcription factor (MiTF) and SOX-10, which are nuclear markers, allow more precise quantification to be performed (Fig. 12.2) (Ruben 2015).

Melanocytic Nevus

A nevus is a benign neoplasm characterized by the presence of melanocytic nests and variable numbers of single melanocytes, primarily located in the nail matrix and possibly in the hyponychium and/or ventral portion of the proximal nail fold (Ruben 2015; André et al. 2013; Fernandez-Flores et al. 2014). The nests often consist of large epithelioid melanocytes, are usually scarce, and are rare in the nail bed (Fig. 12.3). Intense melanocytic hyperplasia with confluent nests rarely occurs (André et al. 2013).

When the nail unit is affected, junctional nevus usually occurs. Compound nevi may display nests that are horizontally contoured (Fig. 12.4). Congenital, blue, and Spitz nevi are other forms of presentation (Ruben 2015; André et al. 2013; Fernandez-Flores et al. 2014). Melanoma is an important differential diagnosis; however, certain characteristics suggest the diagnosis of a nevus. For example, the presence of junctional nests, mild and focal stromal lymphocytic infiltrate, and the absence of or mild pagetoid spread and cellular atypia (Fernandez-Flores et al. 2014; Tan et al. 2007). Some authors use the expression "atypical melanocytic hyperplasia" when only scattered, occasional, atypical melanocytes are seen (Fernandez-Flores et al. 2014; Perrin 2013).

The melanocytic nevus is considered the most common form of melanonychia in children, and in this group, histological features may be unusual, making the diagnosis difficult. Some degree of pleomorphism and inflammatory processes in the dermis may occur; however, no confluence of atypical melanocytes is observed (Ruben 2015).

Distinguishing between some lentigines or nevi and early melanomas in situ is particularly difficult; therefore, the histopathological analysis should be meticulous and – when necessary – an immunostain should be performed. SHMB-45, Ki-67, HMB-45, Melan-A, and S100 can be used (Ruben 2015).

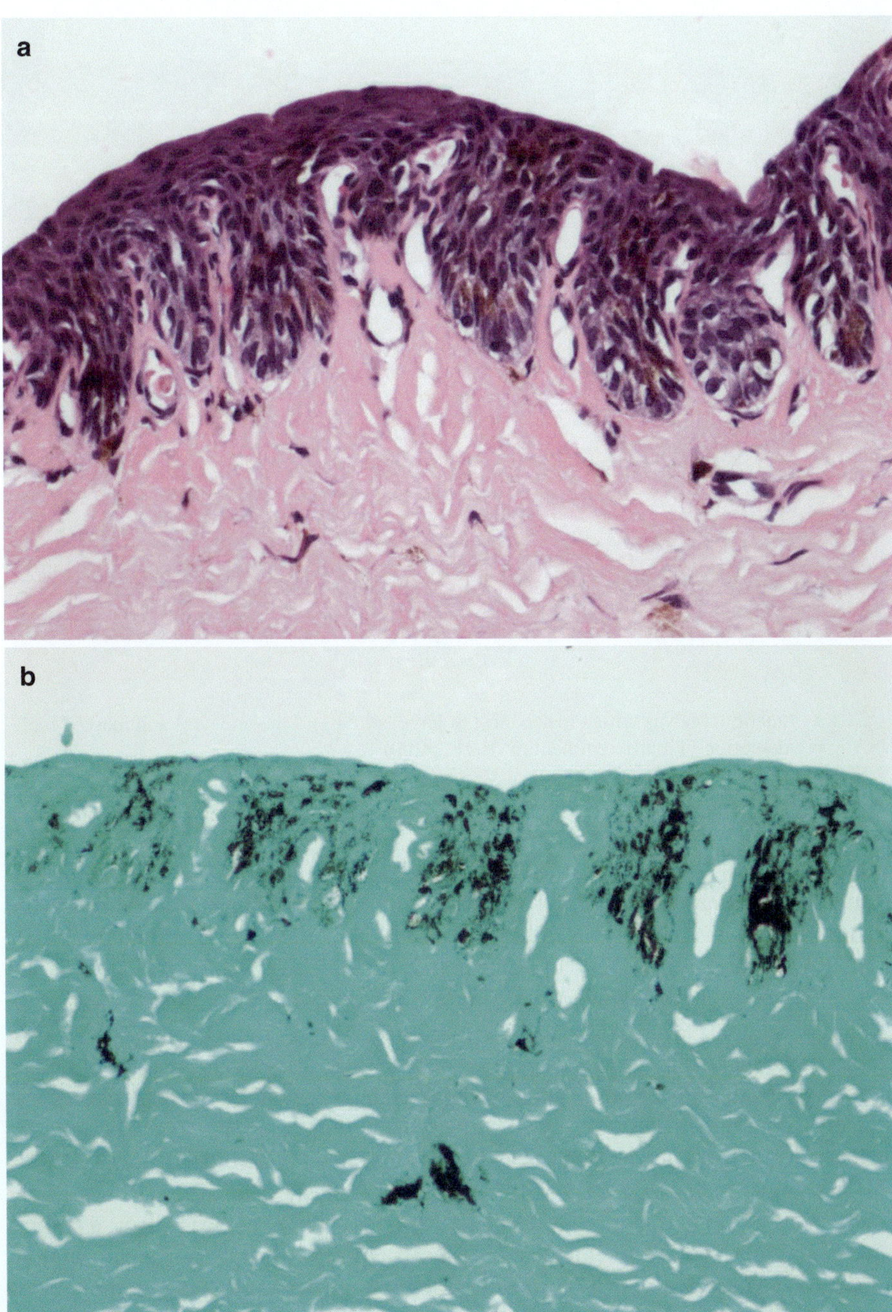

Fig. 12.2 (**a**) Lentiginous nevus (lentigo) with basal melanocytic proliferation accompanied by rete ridges elongation and melanocytic pigmentation of the matrix epithelium (H&E, ×200). (**b**) Fontana–Masson stain highlighting the melanocytic proliferation and pigmentation of the matrix epithelium (×200)

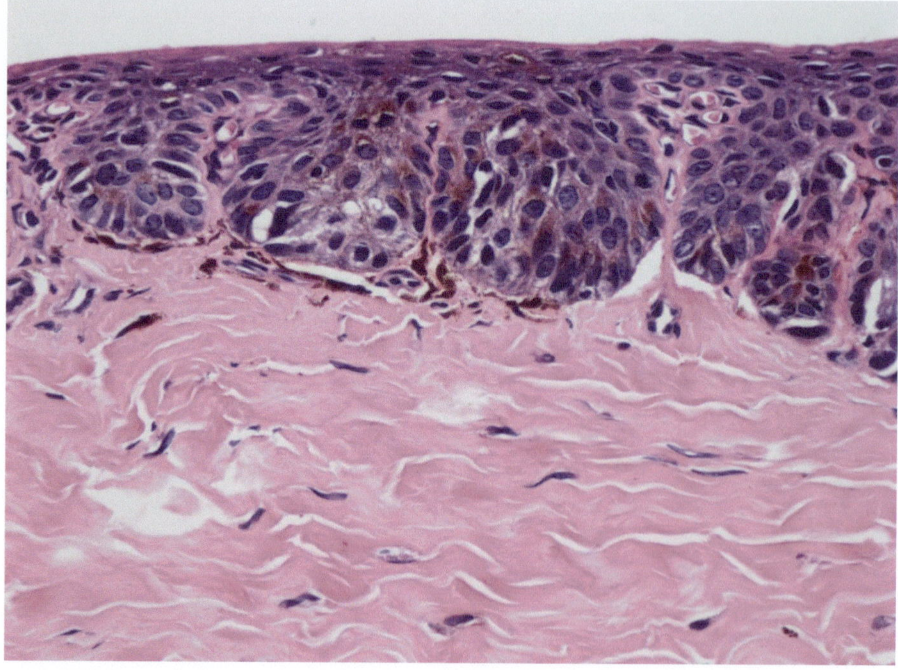

Fig. 12.3 Junctional nevus with a matrix nest of large epithelioid melanocytes and marked melanocytic pigmentation in matrix epithelium (H&E, ×200)

Melanoma

Usually, nail apparatus melanoma originates from the nail matrix as this area has the highest density of melanocytes of the nail unit (André et al. 2013; Fernandez-Flores et al. 2014; Shin and Jang 2014). After that, it can spread to the proximal fold, nail bed, and hyponychium. However, it can start at any of these locations (André et al. 2013; Fernandez-Flores et al. 2014). When originating in the nail matrix, the most common presentation is melanonychia. Otherwise, if originating in the nail bed, it appears as a subungual nodule and onycholysis. Histologically, in situ lesions show an increased number of melanocytes with atypia at the basal layer. Nuclear atypia is moderate and focal in the early stages in addition to pagetoid infiltration. Also, single atypical melanocytes are more frequent than nests (Fig. 12.5) (Ruben 2015; André et al. 2013; Fernandez-Flores et al. 2014). As the lesion progresses, a confluence of single atypical melanocytes forms nests with prominent atypia and pagetoid infiltration (André et al. 2013; Fernandez-Flores et al. 2014). Recently, lymphocytes infiltrating the tumor have been reported to be a diagnostic clue (André et al. 2013).

Nail apparatus melanoma grows radially in the early stages (Shin and Jang 2014; Tan et al. 2007; Izumi et al. 2008). It is considered invasive when atypical

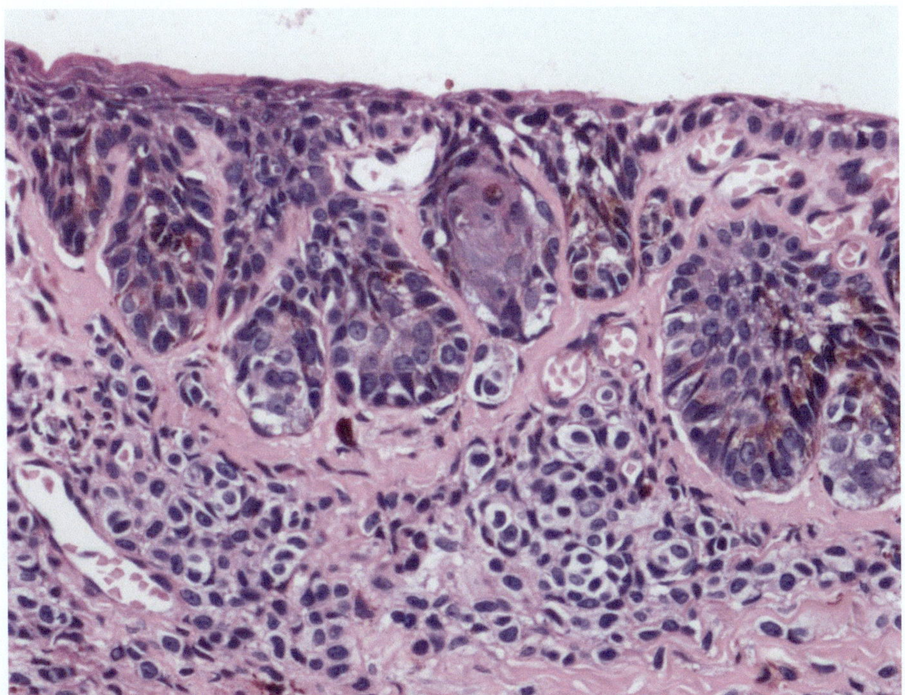

Fig. 12.4 Compound nevus with matrix nest of large epithelioid melanocytes and nevus cells in the superficial corium (H&E, ×200)

melanocytes infiltrate the dermis (Shin and Jang 2014; Tan et al. 2007; Izumi et al. 2008). Clark level and Breslow thickness are more difficult to assess because the unique anatomy of the nail unit (Ruben 2015; André et al. 2013; Fernandez-Flores et al. 2014; Shin and Jang 2014). Indeed, the thickness of the epidermis varies for each region of the nail unit (André et al. 2013; Fernandez-Flores et al. 2014; Shin and Jang 2014). Therefore, the degree of dermal invasion may be different depending on where the measurement is taken. Additionally, as the granular layer is mostly absent in the nail matrix and the nail bed, identifying the Breslow index may be very difficult. On the other hand, it is important to consider that the subcutaneous layer is very thin or absent and it is not easy to recognize the border between the papillary and reticular dermis (André et al. 2013; Shin and Jang 2014). For these reasons, establishing the Clark level may also be a problem (André et al. 2013; Shin and Jang 2014). It has been suggested that melanoma reaching the periosteum or invading underlying bone should be classified as Clark level V[2]. For the reasons explained above, when a subungual melanoma is suspected, it is strongly recommended to perform a longitudinal biopsy including all areas of the nail unit.

Finally, because melanoma thickness is the most important prognostic factor, it is necessary to standardize a measure adapted to the special anatomy of the nail unit.

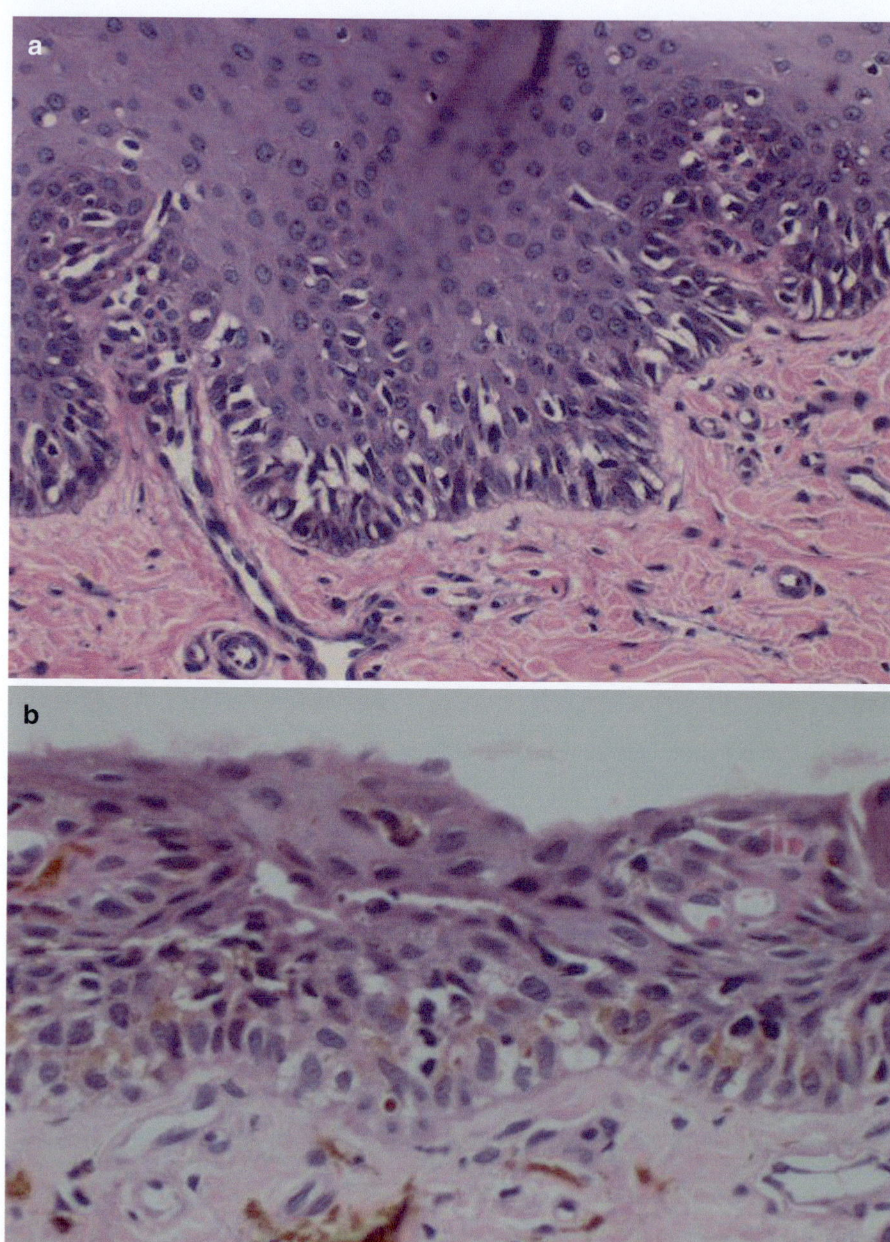

Fig. 12.5 (**a**) In situ lentiginous melanoma showing atypical melanocytes along the basal layer of matrix epithelium, some of them distributed above the basal layer (H&E, ×200). (**b**) In situ melanoma showing atypical melanocytes along the matrix epithelium with some melanophages in the superficial corium (H&E, ×200)

Summary for the Clinician
- The activity and location of melanocytes of the nail matrix are different from those of the normal skin. Pathologists should be familiar with the anatomical features of the nail unit.
- Hypermelanosis (melanocytic activation) appears as an increase in pigment in melanocytes, without any increase in the number of melanocytes.
- A slight to moderate increase in non-atypical – often dendritic – melanocytes in the nail matrix or nail bed, arranged in individual units and located in the basal layer, is observed in cases of lentigo. Mild atypia may occur.
- Melanocytic nests and some single melanocytes in the nail matrix are the main features of melanocytic nevus. Despite melanoma being the main differential diagnosis, some particulars are observed in melanocytic nevi of the nail unit
- Atypical melanocyte proliferation and pagetoid infiltration are common in cases of melanoma of the nail unit. Nests and lymphocyte infiltration can also be seen in the advanced stages.

References

Amin B, Nehal KS, Jungbluth AA, Zaidi B, Brady MS, Coit DC, Zhou Q, Busam KJ. Histologic distinction between subungual lentigo and melanoma. Am J Surg Pathol. 2008;32(6):835–43.

André J, Sass U, Richert B, Theunis A. Nail pathology. Clin Dermatol. 2013;31(5):526–39.

Fernandez-Flores A, Saeb-Lima M, Martínez-Nova A. Histopathology of the nail unit. Rom J Morphol Embryol. 2014;55(2):235–56.

Izumi M, Ohara K, Hoashi T, et al. Subungual melanoma: histological examination of 50 cases from early stage to bone invasion. J Dermatol. 2008;35:695–703.

Perrin C. Tumors of the nail unit. A review. I. Acquired localized longitudinal melanonychia and erythronychia. Am J Dermatopathol. 2013;35(6):621–36.

Ruben BS. Pigmented lesions of the nail unit. Semin Cutan Med Surg. 2015;34(2):101–8.

Shin H-T, Jang K-T. Histopathological analysis of the progression pattern of subungual melanoma: late tendency of dermal invasion in the nail matrix area. Mod Pathol. 2014;27:1461–14677.

Tan KB, Moncrieff M, Thompson JF, McCarthy SW, Shaw HM, Quinn MJ, Li LX, Crotty KA, Stretch JR, Scolyer RA. Subungual melanoma: a study of 124 cases highlighting features of early lesions, potential pitfalls in diagnosis, and guidelines for histologic reporting. Am J Surg Pathol. 2007;31(12):1902–12.

Treatment of Nail Unit Melanoma

Bertrand Richert

Key Features
- Amputation was considered the rule for nail unit melanoma for decades.
- To date, there have been no guidelines for the treatment of melanoma of the nail unit.
- Several studies have shown that there is no evidence that aggressive amputation is associated with higher survival rates.
- The recent literature offers hints in favor of "functional" excision as management of nail unit melanoma in situ and more distal amputation for invasive melanoma.

Introduction

Nail unit melanomas (NUMs) are not more aggressive than other melanomas of similar depth (Patterson and Helwig 1980; Haneke 2012). The poor prognosis of NUMs is linked to the delay in their diagnosis. This delay may be attributed to both the patient, who does not suspect the possibility of cancer at that site – only one-third of patients with longitudinal melanonychia seek medical advice (Thai et al. 2001) – and the low accuracy (46–55%) of physicians making an accurate diagnosis (Di Chiacchio et al. 2010). The latter is made at a late stage, when the lesion has a high Breslow index (Bristow et al. 2010). The 5-year survival rate has been directly linked to the thickness of the tumor: 88% for a Breslow thickness less than 2.5 mm and only 40% for a thickness greater than 2.5 mm (Banfield and Dawber 1999).

B. Richert, MD, PhD
Dermatology Department, Brugmann – Saint Pierre – Queen Fabiola University Hospitals, Université Libre de Bruxelles, Place Van Gehuchten 4, 1020 Brussels, Belgium
e-mail: Bertrand.Richert@chu-brugmann.be

© Springer International Publishing Switzerland 2017
N. Di Chiacchio, A. Tosti (eds.), *Melanonychias*,
DOI 10.1007/978-3-319-44993-7_13

Until now, early diagnosis and excision of the tumor was the only treatment known to increase survival (Thai et al. 2001). To date, there have been no guidelines for the treatment of melanoma of the nail unit.

Diffusion Treatments

The worldwide surgical treatment for NUMs has traditionally been to amputate the digit at the most proximal interphalangeal joint. It was thought to be the best means of preventing recurrence and deadly metastasis. The rationale for amputation was never based on scientific evidence, but on the idea that aggressive surgery was adequate for what was thought to be an aggressive tumor (Cochran et al. 2014). This conclusion comes from a publication by Dasgupta and Brasfield (1965) demonstrating that patients, of a series of 34, who underwent distal amputation did not survive 5 years, compared with patients who benefited from more proximal surgery. However, at any time the depth of the lesion was mentioned and half of the patients were described as having "advanced" disease". Amputation was then considered to be the gold standard treatment for NUMs, confirming what was stated a century earlier by Hutchinson (1886), who wrote that "early amputation is demanded." These two studies with poor clinical evidence have historically guided the surgical treatment of NUMs, and authors continued to advocate aggressive amputation (Patterson and Helwig 1980; Papachristou and Fortner 1982; Slingluff et al. 1990; Pack and Oropeza 1967; Leppard et al. 1974; Paladugu et al. 1983; Gutman et al. 1985; Takematsu et al. 1985; Daly et al. 1987; Rigby and Briggs 1992; Quinn et al. 1996) until the 2000s, when several studies concluded that proximal amputation (metacarpophalangeal joint) versus distal amputation (proximal or distal interphalangeal joint) did not have a significant impact on overall survival (Heaton et al. 1994; Slingluff et al. 1990; Finley et al. 1994; Thai et al. 2001; Martin et al. 2011). None of them are randomized or prospective studies and available scientific data come from retrospective studies, mostly with a bias in the choice of the treatment, as more distal amputation was performed in less invasive lesions, whereas for a higher Breslow index, a more proximal amputation was chosen. Level of evidence was mainly 3 or 4; one study even level 5 (Cochran et al. 2014). To our knowledge, Park et al. was the first to treat NUM patients without amputation but with "local excision", paving the way to less aggressive management of NUMs (Park et al. 1992). In the largest subungual melanoma study ever published, they showed that distal amputation or local excision did not compromise the overall survival of these patients compared with those undergoing more proximal disarticulation. The seven patients treated with "local excision" had no recurrence. Park et al. concluded that because nearly 70% of these tumors arose on the thumb or hallux, adequate clearance should be obtained and less radical excision should be performed to maintain maximal function. He was the precursor of so-called "functional surgery".

For about 10 years, the literature offered hints in favor of "functional" excision as management of NUMs in situ. (Moehrle et al. 2003; Duarte et al. 2010; Lazar et al. 2005; Sureda et al. 2011; Chow et al. 2013). Moehrle et al. compared NUM treatment in 62 patients, with varying thickness (Breslow 1–4 mm, mean 1.68 mm). Thirty-one cases were treated with conservative "functional" surgery (removal of the whole nail unit with resection of the corona unguicularis) and 31 with distal phalanx amputation. They did not find any significant difference regarding recurrence or survival between the two groups, which reached 92% at 5 years (Moehrle et al. 2003). Sureda et al. treated a series of seven patients with NUM in situ or microinvasive (up to 0.2 mm) with wide local excision and had a 100% survival rate at 45 months (Sureda et al. 2011). Neczyporenko et al. have published the first largest series of patients with only NUM in situ and followed them for the longest period (mean duration 65.5 months; range 5–157 months). All patients underwent complete nail unit removal with 6-mm security margins around the anatomical boundaries of the nail. All 11 patients survived, but two recurred very late, after 7 and 11 years respectively. A more recent study on 50 patients with in situ and less than 0.5 mm melanoma confirms the excellent results of functional surgery (Nakamura et al. 2015). The recurrences were treated by distal amputation (Neczyporenko et al. 2014). One publication reported less positive results for conservative surgery: four NUMs in situ out of six treated by local excision required further amputation, owing to positive margins in three patients and local recurrence in one (Cohen et al. 2008). However, safety margins were variable or not well defined ("wide," "generous"), and no correlation between margins and recurrence rate was mentioned.

Several case series have reported Mohs surgery, with encouraging results (Banfield et al. 1999; Brodland 2001).

History

As it was demonstrated that aggressive amputation did not change the prognosis of the patient, the current trend is toward a much more conservative approach to the management of NUMs. However, the literature does not provide a high enough level of evidence, and further studies, especially prospective studies, are still needed.

Physiopathology

Although trauma has often been mentioned as a potential causative factor, no link could be established with certainty (Möhrle and Häfner 2002). Ultraviolet radiation is not responsible either as the nail plate acts as a barrier (Stern et al. 2011), the matrix area where the melanoma arises is not directly exposed to sunlight, and the similar occurrence of NUMs in dark- and fair-skinned races suggests that pigmentation might not be protective (Thai et al. 2001). NUM genetics appear to be peculiar, as far as the expression of *BRAF*, *NRAS*, and *KIT* genes is concerned. With regard to the rarely detected *BRAF* mutations and the more frequent mutations in the *KIT* gene, NUMs appear to be similar to acral melanomas (Dika et al. 2013).

The thumb and the great toenail are most frequently affected (Tan et al. 2007), probably because of the larger proportion of the matrix on these digits (Banfield and Dawber 1999). NUMs mainly arise from the nail matrix, but also from the bed and/or the lateral folds, structures containing melanocytes (Koga et al. 2011). In three-quarters of the cases, NUMs develop in the matrix and the first symptom is longitudinal melanonychia (Ishihara et al. 1993). In 30% of the cases, NUMs arise from the nail bed and present as a nodule, pigmented or not, ulceration with bleeding, isolated fold pigmentation, unexplained monodactylic paronychia or a partial destruction of the nail plate (Tosti et al. 2009). The clinician should remember that about 20–30% of NUMs are amelanotic (Thai et al. 2001). It is even more treacherous when it manifests as monodactylic onychorrhexis (André et al. 2010).

Treatment

Treatment for NUMs is surgical. Increasingly, authors report treatment of in situ and micro-invasive NUMs (Breslow <0.5 mm) by "en-bloc" removal of the nail unit, which seems reasonable according to the published data, even if there is not a high level of evidence (Thai et al. 2001; Di Chiacchio et al. 2010). There are three main issues in the management of NUMs in situ:

1. The certainty that the melanoma is really in situ. The biopsy of suspected longitudinal melanonychia should always be excisional and not incisional. The whole specimen may then be examined by the pathologist on serial cuts, to ensure that the melanoma remains in situ throughout the tumor.
2. The width of the lateral margins. It has been demonstrated, using genomic hybridization and fluorescent in situ hybridization, that melanocytic cells with genetic amplifications were detected in histopathologically normal skin, with a mean extension of 6.1 mm (in situ melanomas) and 4.5 mm (invasive melanomas) beyond the histopathological margin. Genetic profiling of these cells indicated that they represent an early phase of disease preceding melanoma in situ. The melanoma cells extend significantly into seemingly normal skin. These cells provide a plausible explanation for the tendency of certain melanoma types to recur locally, despite apparently having undergone complete excision (North et al. 2008). This may explain why in studies acknowledging wide local excision of 5–10 mm, the recurrence rate is almost nil for in situ melanomas.
3. The thickness of the deep margin. A recent study on cadavers evaluated the distance from the lowest base of the nail matrix to the phalangeal bony surface. The average distance of all digits was 0.90 mm, and the shortest distance among the measured specimens was 0.27 mm (Kim et al. 2011). Thus, some soft tissue may remain adherent to the bone after en-bloc ablation of the nail unit, because of the paucity of the subungual soft tissue between the tumor and the bone beneath the nail apparatus. Only very skilled surgeons are able to perform the so-called "skeletization" (Fig. 13.1). This is why Chow proposed to remove a 1-mm horizontal slice of the underlying bone using an oscillating saw (Chow et al. 2013). This ensures better control of the deep margin and ensures preservation of the length of the digit. To be efficient, this procedure should involve the proximal bony phalanx underlying the matrix, without harming the extensor tendon.

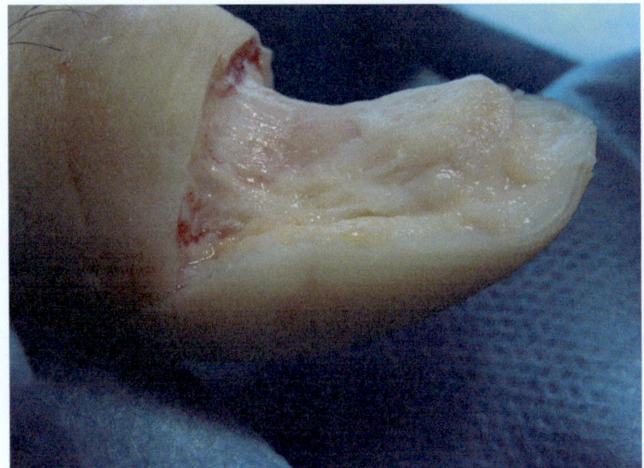

Fig. 13.1 Removal of the nail unit skimming the bone gives rise to "skeletization." Note how far the incision extends laterally to ensure complete removal of the lateral horns of the matrix

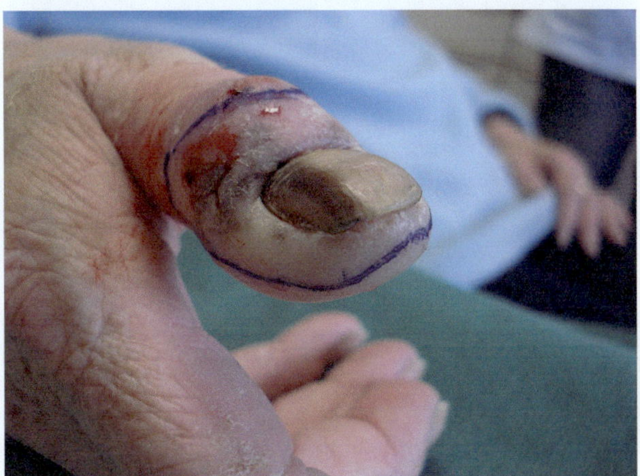

Fig. 13.2 Note that the incision line extends 6 mm beyond the Hutchinson's sign

Thus, surgical treatment of melanoma in situ should include en-bloc excision of the nail unit, with at least 6-mm margins around the anatomical boundaries of the nail unit (including the lateral horns of the matrix), skimming the periosteum, leading to a real "skeletization." If the surgeon can achieve it, removal of a slice of the most superficial part of the bone should be performed. In the presence of any existing Hutchinson's sign, the excision lines should extend 6 mm beyond the borders of the pigmentation (Fig. 13.2). This sign characterizes the horizontal spread of the disease. Closure may be achieved by either secondary intention or full-thickness grafting (Lazar et al. 2005; High et al. 2004; Rayatt et al. 2007; Duarte et al. 2010; Sureda et al. 2011). The author prefers secondary intention for toes, as the graft may suffer because of footwear and accidental shock (Fig. 13.3). For fingers, grafting gives a more aesthetic aspect: there is no retraction, the shape of the graft is similar to that of a nail, and the graft offers padding to the underlying bone (Fig. 13.4), as opposed to secondary intention healing, where the superficial tissues adhere to the

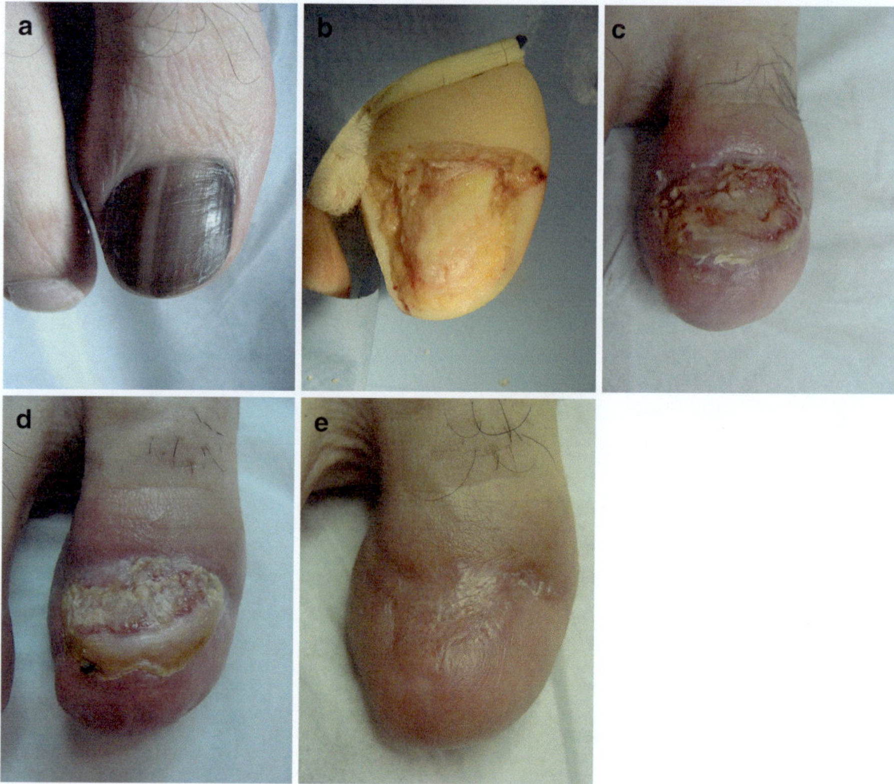

Fig. 13.3 (**a–e**) Secondary intention healing for a melanoma in situ in the great toenail

bone (Fig. 13.5). Some authors have utilized artificial dermis for closure (Hayashi et al. 2012).

The recent development of intraoperative reflectance confocal microscopy examination of the nail matrix has enabled one-step surgical management of in situ or minimally invasive melanomas, reducing dramatically the duration of postoperative disability (Debarbieux et al. 2012).

For invasive NUMs, as there is no evidence that aggressive amputation is associated with higher survival rates, amputation should be aimed at retaining the greatest function possible (Nguyen et al. 2013).

Sentinel lymph node biopsy (SLNB) helps to stage the cancer and dictates further adjunctive therapy. Although it was debated for a long time, a recent study has shown that the merit of SLNB could be confined to patients with thick (>1 mm) or ulcerated acral lentiginous melanomas. This meets the 2009 American Joint Committee on Cancer (AJCC) recommendations (Balch et al. 2009; Ito et al. 2015).

Isolated limb perfusion does not affect overall survival rates (Heaton et al. 1994).

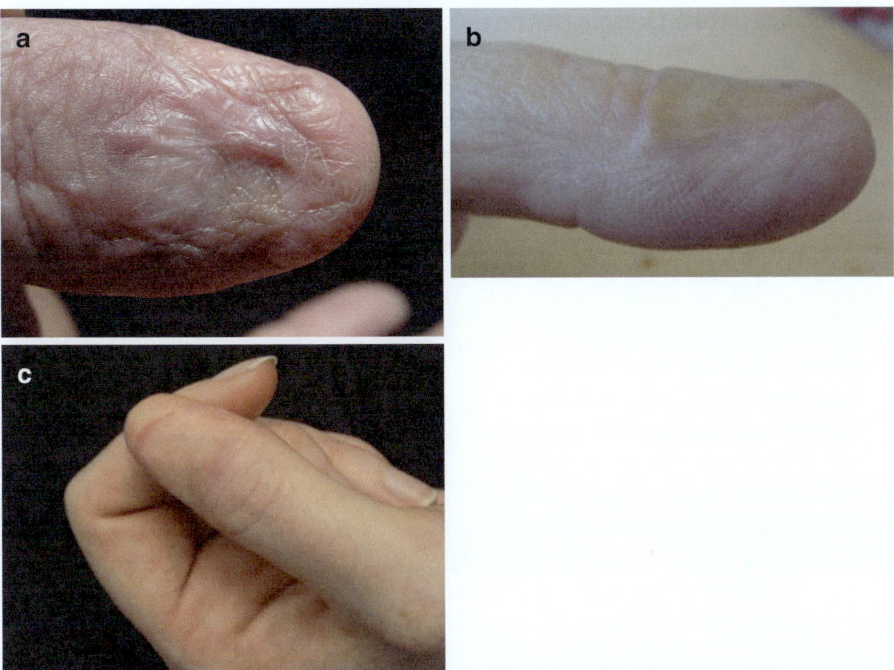

Fig. 13.4 (**a–c**) Full-thickness grafting after "en-bloc" removal of the nail unit. Note the cosmetic aspect and the padding of skin over the bone

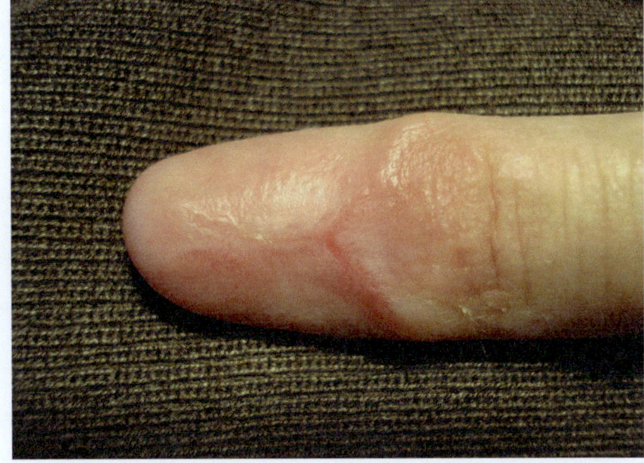

Fig. 13.5 Secondary intention healing. Note the adherence of the skin to the bone

Outlook: Future Developments

Acral lentiginous melanomas may have different oncogenetic pathways. Knowledge of the gene expression profile may have important implications in disease management and treatment, thanks to the development of new drugs, such as *KIT*- and *MAPK*-targeted kinase inhibitors (Hocker et al. 2008). For example, it has been recently shown that *TERT* gene amplification is associated with poor outcome in acral lentiginous melanoma (Diaz et al. 2014).

> **Summary for the Clinician**
> The studies in the literature involving amputation for the treatment of NUMs did not prove any significant benefit with regard to prognosis and/or survival rate over the more conservative treatment of excision. The level of evidence of the vast majority of articles on the treatment of NUMs is relatively poor. However, the collective data suggest that NUMs in situ might be treated adequately with wide local excision. For invasive melanoma, the level of amputation should be guided by a balance between the thickness of the tumor and the conservation of function. There is still a lack of randomized prospective studies.

References

André J, Moulonguet I, Goettmann-Bonvallot S. In situ amelanotic melanoma of the nail unit mimicking lichen planus: report of 3 cases. Arch Dermatol. 2010;146(4):418–21.

Balch CM, Gershenwald JE, Soong S-J, Thompson JF, Atkins MB, Byrd DR, et al. Final version of 2009 AJCC melanoma staging and classification. J Clin Oncol. 2009;27(36):6199–206.

Banfield CC, Dawber RP. Nail melanoma: a review of the literature with recommendations to improve patient management. Br J Dermatol. 1999;141(4):628–32.

Banfield CC, Dawber RP, Walker NP, Stables GI, Zeina B, Schomberg K. Mohs micrographic surgery for the treatment of in situ nail apparatus melanoma: a case report. J Am Acad Dermatol. 1999;40(1):98–9.

Bristow IR, de Berker DA, Acland KM, Turner RJ, Bowling J. Clinical guidelines for the recognition of melanoma of the foot and nail unit. J Foot Ankle Res. 2010;3:25.

Brodland DG. The treatment of nail apparatus melanoma with Mohs micrographic surgery. Dermatol Surg. 2001;27(3):269–73.

Chow WTH, Bhat W, Magdub S, Orlando A. In situ subungual melanoma: digit salvaging clearance. J Plast Reconstr Aesthet Surg. 2013;66(2):274–6.

Cochran AM, Buchanan PJ, Bueno RA, Neumeister MW. Subungual melanoma: a review of current treatment. Plast Reconstr Surg. 2014;134(2):259–73.

Cohen T, Busam KJ, Patel A, Brady MS. Subungual melanoma: management considerations. Am J Surg. 2008;195(2):244–8.

Daly JM, Berlin R, Urmacher C. Subungual melanoma: a 25-year review of cases. J Surg Oncol. 1987;35(2):107–12.

Dasgupta T, Brasfield R. Subungual melanoma: 25-year review of cases. Ann Surg. 1965;161:545–52.

Debarbieux S, Hospod V, Depaepe L, Balme B, Poulalhon N, Thomas L. Perioperative confocal microscopy of the nail matrix in the management of in situ or minimally invasive subungual melanomas. Br J Dermatol. 2012;167(4):828–36.

Di Chiacchio N, Hirata SH, Enokihara MY, Michalany NS, Fabbrocini G, Tosti A. Dermatologists' accuracy in early diagnosis of melanoma of the nail matrix. Arch Dermatol. 2010;146(4):382–7.

Diaz A, Puig-Butillé JA, Muñoz C, Costa D, Díez A, Garcia-Herrera A, et al. TERT gene amplification is associated with poor outcome in acral lentiginous melanoma. J Am Acad Dermatol. 2014;71(4):839–41.

Dika E, Altimari A, Patrizi A, Gruppioni E, Fiorentino M, Piraccini BM, et al. KIT, NRAS, and BRAF mutations in nail apparatus melanoma. Pigment Cell Melanoma Res. 2013;26(5):758–60.

Duarte AF, Correia O, Barros AM, Azevedo R, Haneke E. Nail matrix melanoma in situ: conservative surgical management. Dermatology (Basel). 2010;220(2):173–5.

Finley 3rd RK, Driscoll DL, Blumenson LE, Karakousis CP. Subungual melanoma: an eighteen-year review. Surgery. 1994;116(1):96–100.

Gutman M, Klausner JM, Inbar M, Skornick Y, Baratz M, Rozin RR. Acral (volar-subungual) melanoma. Br J Surg. 1985;72(8):610–3.

Haneke E. Ungual melanoma – controversies in diagnosis and treatment. Dermatol Ther. 2012;25(6):510–24.

Hayashi K, Uhara H, Koga H, Okuyama R, Saida T. Surgical treatment of nail apparatus melanoma in situ: the use of artificial dermis in reconstruction. Dermatol Surg. 2012;38(4):692–4.

Heaton KM, el-Naggar A, Ensign LG, Ross MI, Balch CM. Surgical management and prognostic factors in patients with subungual melanoma. Ann Surg. 1994;219(2):197–204.

High WA, Quirey RA, Guillén DR, Munõz G, Taylor RS. Presentation, histopathologic findings, and clinical outcomes in 7 cases of melanoma in situ of the nail unit. Arch Dermatol. 2004;140(9):1102–6.

Hocker TL, Singh MK, Tsao H. Melanoma genetics and therapeutic approaches in the 21st century: moving from the benchside to the bedside. J Invest Dermatol. 2008;128(11):2575–95.

Hutchinson J. Melanosis often not black: melanotic whitlow. Br Med J. 1886;1:491–4.

Ito T, Wada M, Nagae K, Nakano-Nakamura M, Nakahara T, Hagihara A, Furue M, Uchi H. Acral lentiginous melanoma: who benefits from sentinel lymph node biopsy? J Am Acad Dermatol. 2015;72(1):71–7.

Ishihara Y, Matsumoto K, Kawachi S, Saida T. Detection of early lesions of "ungual" malignant melanoma. Int J Dermatol. 1993;32(1):44–7.

Kim JY, Jung HJ, Lee WJ, Kim DW, Yoon GS, Kim D-S, et al. Is the distance enough to eradicate in situ or early invasive subungual melanoma by wide local excision? From the point of view of matrix-to-bone distance for safe inferior surgical margin in Koreans. Dermatology (Basel). 2011;223(2):122–3.

Koga H, Saida T, Uhara H. Key point in dermoscopic differentiation between early nail apparatus melanoma and benign longitudinal melanonychia. J Dermatol. 2011;38(1):45–52.

Lazar A, Abimelec P, Dumontier C. Full thickness skin graft for nail unit reconstruction. J Hand Surg Br. 2005;30(2):194–8.

Leppard B, Sanderson KV, Behan F. Subungual malignant melanoma: difficulty in diagnosis. Br Med J. 1974;1(5903):310–2.

Martin DE, English JC, Goitz RJ. Subungual malignant melanoma. J Hand Surg Am. 2011;36(4):704–7.

Moehrle M, Metzger S, Schippert W, Garbe C, Rassner G, Breuninger H. "Functional" surgery in subungual melanoma. Dermatol Surg. 2003;29(4):366–74.

Möhrle M, Häfner HM. Is subungual melanoma related to trauma? Dermatol (Basel). 2002;204(4):259–61.

Nakamura Y, Ohara K, Kishi A, Teramoto Y, Sato S, Fujisawa Y, Fujimoto M, Otsuka F, Hayashi N, Yamazaki N, Yamamoto A. Effects of non-amputative wide local excision on the local control and prognosis of in situ and invasive subungual melanoma. J Dermatol. 2015;42(9):861–6.

Neczyporenko F, André J, Torosian K, Theunis A, Richert B. Management of in situ melanoma of the nail apparatus with functional surgery: report of 11 cases and review of the literature. J Eur Acad Dermatol Venereol. 2014;28(5):550–7.

Nguyen JT, Bakri K, Nguyen EC, Johnson CH, Moran SL. Surgical management of subungual melanoma: mayo clinic experience of 124 cases. Ann Plast Surg. 2013;71(4):346–54.

North JP, Kageshita T, Pinkel D, LeBoit PE, Bastian BC. Distribution and significance of occult intraepidermal tumor cells surrounding primary melanoma. J Invest Dermatol. 2008;128(8):2024–30.

Pack GT, Oropeza R. Subungual melanoma. Surg Gynecol Obstet. 1967;124(3):571–82.

Paladugu RR, Winberg CD, Yonemoto RH. Acral lentiginous melanoma. A clinicopathologic study of 36 patients. Cancer. 1983;52(1):161–8.

Papachristou DN, Fortner JG. Melanoma arising under the nail. J Surg Oncol. 1982;21(4):219–22.

Park KG, Blessing K, Kernohan NM. Surgical aspects of subungual malignant melanomas. Scott Melanoma Group Ann Surg. 1992;216(6):692–5.

Patterson RH, Helwig EB. Subungual malignant melanoma: a clinical-pathologic study. Cancer. 1980;46(9):2074–87.

Quinn MJ, Thompson JE, Crotty K, McCarthy WH, Coates AS. Subungual melanoma of the hand. J Hand Surg Am. 1996;21(3):506–11.

Rayatt SS, Dancey AL, Davison PM. Thumb subungual melanoma: is amputation necessary? J Plast Reconstr Aesthet Surg. 2007;60(6):635–8.

Rigby HS, Briggs JC. Subungual melanoma: a clinico-pathological study of 24 cases. Br J Plast Surg. 1992;45(4):275–8.

Slingluff CL, Vollmer R, Seigler HF. Acral melanoma: a review of 185 patients with identification of prognostic variables. J Surg Oncol. 1990;45(2):91–8.

Stern DK, Creasey AA, Quijije J, Lebwohl MG. UV-A and UV-B penetration of normal human cadaveric fingernail plate. Arch Dermatol. 2011;147(4):439–41.

Sureda N, Phan A, Poulalhon N, Balme B, Dalle S, Thomas L. Conservative surgical management of subungual (matrix derived) melanoma: report of seven cases and literature review. Br J Dermatol. 2011;165(4):852–8.

Takematsu H, Obata M, Tomita Y, Kato T, Takahashi M, Abe R. Subungual melanoma. A clinico-pathologic study of 16 Japanese cases. Cancer. 1985;55(11):2725–31.

Tan K-B, Moncrieff M, Thompson JF, McCarthy SW, Shaw HM, Quinn MJ, et al. Subungual melanoma: a study of 124 cases highlighting features of early lesions, potential pitfalls in diagnosis, and guidelines for histologic reporting. Am J Surg Pathol. 2007;31(12):1902–12.

Thai KE, Young R, Sinclair RD. Nail apparatus melanoma. Australas J Dermatol. 2001;42(2):71–81.. quiz 82–83

Tosti A, Piraccini BM, de Farias DC. Dealing with melanonychia. Semin Cutan Med Surg. 2009;28(1):49–54.

Index

A
ABCDEF rule, 10, 13, 18–21, 36, 63
Acquired melanonychia, 61
Acral lentiginous melanoma (ALM), 71, 72,
    146–148
Atypical melanocytes, 82, 113, 134, 136, 138
  proliferation of, 80, 81

B
Bacterial stain, enterobacteria, 64, 66
Biopsy technique
  anesthesia, 121
  complications, 129
  dermoscopic examination, 122
  hemostasis, 121, 124
  indications, 120
  intraoperative dermoscopy, 123
  medical history, 121
  melanonychia pigment, 122, 123
  nail avulsion, complete/partial, 123–125
  nail matrix, exposure and visualization,
    123
  nail unit anatomy, 121
  patient positioning, 122
  postprocedural inflammation, 128–129
  preoperative preparation, 121–122
  risk factors, 121–122
  specimen sample, 128
Black onychomycosis, molds, 64, 66
Blue nevi, nail matrix, 3, 41

C
Children, melanonychia in
  Addison's disease, 88
  arsenic intoxication, 88

benign, 87
clinical features, 85, 90–91
dermoscopic features, 85
epidemiology, 86–87
hemochromatosis, 88
incidence, 85
malignancy, 87
melanocyte activation, 87, 89
nail matrix nevi, 91, 92
non-invasive techniques, 86
objective discrimination index, 93
parental anxiety, 93
personal/family history, 87, 94
proliferative process, 90
tangential excision, 94
vitamin B12 deficiency, 88
Congenital nevi, 62

D
Dermatophytes, 11, 98, 99
Dermoscopy of the nail matrix and bed
    (DNMB). *See also* Nail plate
    dermoscopy
  algorithm, 42
  diagnosis, 42
  history, 36
  intraoperative, 36–37
  patterns, LM diagnosis, 37–41
  polarized light dermoscopy, 36
  surgical procedure, 37–38
DOPA-positive melanocytes, 2, 46

E
Epithelial tumors with melanocyte
    population, 64

© Springer International Publishing Switzerland 2017
N. Di Chiacchio, A. Tosti (eds.), *Melanonychias*,
DOI 10.1007/978-3-319-44993-7

F

Fontana–Masson staining, 112, 114, 116, 122, 132, 133
Frictional melanonychia, 6
Fungal melanonychia
    antifungal therapy, 99
    Candida and paronychia, 99, 101
    causative organisms, 98
    dematiaceous fungi, 99
    dermatophyte molds, 98, 99
    due to *Pseudomonas,* 99, 101
    matrix melanocytes, 99
    nondermatophyte molds, 99, 100
    with onycholysis and *Pseudomonas,* 99, 101
    onychomycosis, 98
    polymerase chain reaction, 99
    pyocyanin, 99

H

Hormonal diseases, 64
Hutchinson's sign, 18, 20, 29, 62, 72–75, 80, 90, 122, 142, 145
Hypermelanosis (melanocytic activation), 6, 28, 37, 42, 45–47, 49, 50, 86, 87–89, 111, 112, 114, 131–133
    benign, 12, 13
    causes, 55
    clinical features, 47
    dermatological conditions, 50
    DNMB, 37, 38
    epidemiology, 46
    frictional trauma, 49–50
    histopathology, 132, 133
    history, 46
    iatrogenic causes, 47–48
    local trauma, 49
    nail plate dermoscopy, 29–31
    nonmelanocytic tumors, 52–53
    onychotillomania, 49, 50
    pathogenic causes, 51
    physiologic/racial, 46–48
    post-inflammatory bands, 50, 51
    systemic pathological conditions, 51–52

I

Inflammatory nail diseases, 64

J

Junctional nevus, 91, 92, 134, 136

L

Lateral longitudinal nail biopsy/excision, 127
Laugier–Hunziker–Baran syndrome, 62
Laugier–Hunziker syndrome, 52, 87
Lentiginous nevus (lentigo)
    DNMB, 37, 39
    histopathology, 134, 135
    nail matrix
        causes, 58
        clinical pattern, 58, 59, 61
        history, 58
        periungual pigmentation, 58, 59
        prevalence, 58
        significance, 61
        silver nitrate stain, 64, 67
        in thumb nail, 58, 59
        treatment, 67
    nail plate dermoscopy, 31, 32
Lentigo simplex, 12
Limb perfusion isolation, 147
Longitudinal matrix excision, 127–128
Longitudinal melanonychia (LM), 61, 128
    ABCDEF rule, 10
    aging, 13
    benign melanocytic activation, 12, 13
    brown–black pigment, 9
    in children, 21
    clinical examination, 16–18
    color, 73–74
    diagnosis, 9–10, 26
    epidemiology, 10
    frictional melanonychia, 6
    histopathology, 10
    history, 13, 14, 74
    incidence, 6
    lentigines and nevi, 12
    limitations, clinical evaluation, 20–21
    malignant conditions, 12
    medications, 10, 14–15, 15
    melanocyte activation, 87, 89
    nail dystrophy, 74
    patient history, 13–16
    physical examination, 10
    pigmented bands, 15
    progression, 72, 73
    shape, 73
    social and family histories, 10
    width, 72–73

M
Matrix nevus
    causes, 58
    clinical pattern, 58, 60
    diagnosis, 63–64
    history, 58
    prevalence, 58
    significance, 61
    silver nitrate stain, 64, 67
    treatment, 67
Melanic nail pigmentation, 54
Melanocytes
    activation (*see* Hypermelanosis)
    amelanotic, 11
    benign activation, 12, 13
    characteristics, 3–4
    count, 2
    dendrites, 3
    density measurement, 2
    diagnostic accuracy, 4
    epidermal layers, 2, 3
    histology, 2
    history, 2
    hyperplasia, 13, 21, 27, 28,
        36, 42, 86–87, 93, 111–112,
        123, 134
    melanosome-related proteins, 3
    monoclonal antibody HMB45, 3
    of nail, cell population, 1
    proliferation, malignant, 131
    quantification methods, 2
Melanocytic nevi, 12–13, 37,
        62, 85, 93
Melanoma
    in children, 86, 87, 91–93
    functional, 64
    nail matrix
        DNMB, 41
        histopathology, 136–138
        nail plate dermoscopy, 33, 34
Melanonychia. *See also specific terms*
    characteristics, 72–75
    in children (*see* Children,
        melanonychia in)
    functional, 64
    histopathology, 131–138
    in nail nevus, 113, 114
Melanosome, 3, 46
    related proteins, 3
Melanotic macules, 16, 132
Micro-Hutchinson sign, 29, 61, 76, 77
Modified benzidine stain, 114, 117

N
Nail apparatus lesions, 132, 136–138
Nail avulsion, complete/partial, 123–125
Nail clippings, 61, 64, 99, 104, 112, 114, 115
Nail dyschromia, 5
Nail lichen planus, 15
Nail matrix
    blue nevus, 41
    melanocytes (*see* Melanocytes)
    melanomas, 33, 34
    nevus of, 32, 33
Nail matrix nevi
    in children
        acquired, 91
        clinical features, 91
        congenital, 91
        dermoscopic patterns, 91
        histopathology, 92
        LM, 87, 88, 90, 92
        melanocytic proliferation, 86, 87
    DNMB, 37, 39, 40
    nail plate dermoscopy, 32, 33
Nail plate dermoscopy
    clinical features, 26
    distal streaks, 34
    free edge examination, 28
    globular patterns, 34, 35
    melanin, 111
    nail pigmentation, algorithm, 27, 28
    patterns, LM diagnosis, 29–34
    periungual area, 28–29
    periungual hemorrhages, 34
    polarized and nonpolarized devices, 26
    surface patterns, 27
    ultrasound gel, 26, 27
Nail plate pigmentation
    age, 55
    dermatoscopic findings, 53
    diagnostic algorithm, 54–55
    hemorrhage, 112, 114, 117
    histological features, 112–117
    melanin, 111
    melanocytic activation, 111
    neoplastic causes, 112
    patient evaluation, 53
    physical examination, 53
Nail surgery, 123
Nail unit melanomas (NUMs)
    amputation, aggressive, 143
    anatomy, 132
    diffusion treatments, 142–143
    full-thickness grafting, 145

Nail unit melanomas (NUMs) (*cont.*)
   functional surgery, 143
   gene expression profile, 148
   history, 143
   margin thickness, 144
   Mohs surgery, 143
   nail unit removal, 143
   physiopathology, 143–144
   prognosis, 141
   surgical treatment, 142, 144
   survival rate, 141
   treatment
      en-bloc excision, 144, 147
      intraoperative reflectance confocal
         microscopy, 146
      melanoma in situ, 144, 145
      phalangeal bony surface, 144
      secondary intention healing, 145,
         146–147
      skeletization, 144, 145
Neoplasms, 3–4, 18, 46, 99, 107–108,
   116, 134
Nevoid nail melanoma in childhood, 91
Nondermatophytes, 11, 100
Non-melanocytic melanonychia
   algorithm, 108, 109
   diagnosis, 97, 108
   epidemiology, 98
   fungal (*see* Fungal melanonychia)
   lesions, 132
   signs, 108

O
Onychomatricoma, 64, 65
Onychomycosis
   molds, 64, 66
   nail plate dermoscopy, 35
   pigmentation
      fungi and molds, 113
      nail unit epithelium, 113, 115
      superficial, 113, 116
Onychopapilloma, 64, 65, 108, 109
Onychotillomania, 54

P
Peutz–Jeghers syndrome, 52, 87
Pigmented Bowen disease, 64
   exogenous, 10–11
   nail plate dermoscopy, 35

Pigmented onychomycosis
   dematiaceous fungi and molds, 113
   nail unit epithelium, 113, 115
   superficial, 113, 116
Post-traumatic single-digit black onychomycosis, 64, 66
Pseudo-Hutchinson's sign, 28, 29, 87, 88, 122

S
Sentinel lymph node biopsy (SLNB), 146, 147
Staining, 105–107
   bacterial, enterobacteria, 64, 66
   Fontana–Masson staining, 112, 116
   modified benzidine, 114
   silver nitrate, 64, 67
Subungual hematoma
   due to friction, 64, 65
   hallux, 11, 12
   nail plate dermoscopy, 34, 35
Subungual hemorrhage, 15, 35, 102, 105,
   107, 120
Subungueal melanoma (SUM)
   acrolentiginous type, 13
   algorithmic approach, 79
   ALM, 71
   biopsy types, 78, 79
   conservative surgical treatment, 83
   dermoscopy, 76–78
   diagnosis, 75, 76
   epidemiology, 10, 72
   history, 10, 14, 72
   in situ, 80–81
   invasive, 81, 82
   LM, 9–10
   location, 74
   melanocyte count, 2
   melanonychia characteristics, 72–75
   with nail dystrophy, 74–75
   SLNB, 83
   treatment, 81–83
Syndrome-associated melanonychia, 52

T
Tangential shave nail matrix biopsy, 125–126
Three-millimeter punch biopsy excision,
   126–127
Total melanonychia, 47, 72, 73, 87, 89
Touraine syndrome, 52
Transverse melanonychia, 47, 48

Trap-door avulsion technique, 124, 125
Trauma
    caution, 104
    chronic, 102, 103
    habit tic dystrophy, 102, 103
    matrix melanocytes, 104–105
    melanocyte activation, 102
    nail clipping, 103, 104
    onycholytic nail, 103, 104
    onychopapilloma, 104, 105
    splinter hemorrhages, 104
    subungual blood, 102
    subungual hemorrhage, 102, 104, 105, 109
Tyrosinase-related protein-1 (TRP-1), 3

MIX
Papier aus verantwortungsvollen Quellen
Paper from responsible sources
FSC® C105338

www.fsc.org
FSC

If you have any concerns about our products,
you can contact us on
ProductSafety@springernature.com

In case Publisher is established outside the EU,
the EU authorized representative is:
Springer Nature Customer Service Center GmbH
Europaplatz 3, 69115 Heidelberg, Germany

Printed by Libri Plureos GmbH
in Hamburg, Germany